WHY DO YOU OVEREAT?

WHEN ALL YOU WANT IS TO BE SLIM

I can be contacted at
www.whydoyouovereat.com.

This book is dedicated to my husband, Andy.
He knows why!

Zoë Harcombe

Published by Accent Press Ltd,
Pembroke Dock, Pembrokeshire.
www.accentpress.co.uk

Printed in the UK by
Clays Ltd, St Ives Plc.

Cover design by Rachel Loosmore
Accent Press Ltd.

ISBN 0954489993

The advice offered in this book, although based on the author's
experience and over twenty years of research, is not intended to
be a substitute for the advice of your personal physician.
Always consult a medical practitioner before embarking on any
diet. Neither the author nor the publisher can be held
responsible for any loss or claim arising from the use or misuse
of this book.

ACKNOWLEDGEMENTS

Sincere thanks to the following for granting permission to print the quotes in Chapters 9 and 10:

- Dr Robert Buist "*Food Intolerance - What it is & How to cope with it*" (1984)
- Dr Marshall Mandell & Lynne Scanlon "*5-day Allergy Relief System*" (1979)
- Dr Morton Walker & Dr John Parks Trowbridge "*The Yeast Syndrome*" (1986)
- Harper Collins – Dr Keith Mumby "*The Allergy Handbook*" (1988) & Dr Theron Randolph & Ralph Moss "*Allergies - your hidden enemy*" (1981)
- Macmillan – Dr Richard Mackarness "*Not all in the mind*" (1976)
- McGraw-Hill Companies – Shirley Lorenzani "*Candida - a Twentieth Century Disease*" (1986)
- Random House – Elson Haas & Cameron Stauth "*The False Fat Diet*" (2001)

Sincere thanks also to:

Bob & Hazel Cushion, John & Verna Dent, Karen Easter, Anna Milic, Rachel Loosmore and Nick Naysmith.

WHY DO YOU OVEREAT?

WHEN ALL YOU WANT IS TO BE SLIM

"I was so excited just reading the back cover – this was me! I lost 7lb in the first 10 days without feeling hungry at all."

"For the first time in my life I know I will be slim. I have started the programme, I'm not hungry, the cravings have gone and I know how to stop them coming back. The feeling of liberation is indescribable."

"This seems so unfair! I am now at my ideal weight and I love fitting into all my clothes and yet I can eat chocolate, ice-cream, just about anything I want and maintain this weight. I've become a complete cheating connoisseur (as this book explains) and I get away with whatever I can."

"I lost 70lb on this programme. It was easy to follow. I never felt hungry. I could eat out, take lunches to work, go on holiday and carry on with my normal life whilst still losing weight. It is so practical and effective. All my colleagues were asking me how I had lost so much weight and I actually didn't want to tell them. I wanted to keep the secret to myself!"

"I've changed my weighing day to Wednesday and last night I had lost 14.5lb – my first stone!!! This weight loss has been ENTIRELY due to you and your wonderful book. It gave me an understanding and has made this weight loss extremely easy… it is an awesome thought to know that I shall continue to lose weight thanks to minor changes in my diet. So my sincere thanks, it is doing wonders for my self esteem and life has never been so exciting and challenging."

"I always put on weight on holiday but, since following this eating plan, I no longer put on a single pound, even during a fortnight's holiday. With just a couple of small changes to *how* and *when* I eat, I can eat just about anything and still not put on weight. The tiny adjustments I make are hardly any sacrifice and they are more than worth it given the joy of not having to diet when I get back from holiday."

"I started Phase 1 and after 2 days I had lost 5lb. I actually thought the scales were wrong but I got on the next day and I had definitely lost 5lb. I had just finished an 8 week programme with a personal trainer and I didn't lose a single pound and I was so demotivated. Then I tried this for 2 days and lost 5lb. It was incredible!"

"I have been following your diet for the last 4 days and have lost 5lb! It was a real struggle not to eat sweet things but my willpower held out. Am looking forward to starting Phase 2 to see what happens."

"I started your book last night – and finished it a few hours later! You didn't tell me it would be compulsive! I kept reading about all these things that I knew something about and you pieced them altogether. It made so much sense! I don't need to lose more than a couple of pounds but I do need more energy and I'm sure this Candida thing is a big problem for me. Phase 1 here I come!"

"My husband and I have been on Phase 1 for 2 days and I have lost 2lb and he has lost 6! It's not fair. If he ends up lighter than me that's it!"

"I'm on day 3 of Phase 1 and it's going really well. I don't feel as ill as I thought I would, I have been going to bed early to make the evening temptation time shorter but it's worth it 'cos I've lost half a stone already."

"This is the book I should have written!"
(Said by a Nutritionist, Counsellor, Hypnotherapist & Homeopath)

"I've lost 8lb in 4 days! I can't believe it. I didn't even feel ill like the book said I might. I feel great. I did have huge cravings for sugar for the first couple of days but I didn't give in and I'm really glad I didn't."

"I just couldn't wait to call everyone this morning. I was at mum's last night and weighed myself as we don't have scales at home. I knew I'd lost a lot of weight but I found out I've lost 24lb – nearly 2st! In under a month. I just can't believe it. I've been telling everyone (not that I need to because they can see for themselves!) I feel great too – I can't remember feeling better to be honest. Thank you so much for the diet!"

"Thanks for sending me the book but I haven't managed to look at it yet. My PA has nicked it and won't give it back!"

"I lost 5lb in Phase 1 and I've lost 10lb altogether in the first 2 weeks. Everyone at work wants a copy of your book because they hadn't seen me for a week and didn't recognise me when I got back from Dublin! I feel fantastic too – more energy than ever. My skin is so clear – I just look so well – not just slimmer. Thank you so much."

"I feel like I've got a secret that no one else knows – the secret of how to lose weight! I lost 7lb in Phase 1 and a stone in the first 2 weeks. I socialise a lot so I need to 'cheat' when I'm out and this diet actually tells me how to do that. I have my beer and dinner out but I don't go mad. This is just fantastic!"

"I have every one of the conditions in the book and then some. I have been bed ridden for several days in the past few months I have been so ill. Phase 1 nearly finished me off but I knew why I felt so bad. I just kept thinking of the word 'parasite' and it kept me going. I was so determined I didn't know what had come over me. At the end of Phase 1, I felt incredible. I've been waking at 5.30am with an energy I have never known. I feel clear headed. Until I started this plan I could not remember a day when I had not had chocolate and now I haven't had it for weeks. I just don't crave food any more. I'm loving doing things around the house and the garden with all this energy I now have. I can't thank you enough."

"I can't go anywhere without people talking about 'Zoë's diet' – are you on it? Have you seen so-and-so? I've never read a diet book in my life but I'm going to have to read this one!"

"I just love your book. I'm training for a marathon and have always struggled with sugar highs and lows. I'm following the Phase 2 advice and eating the most enormous quantities you can imagine and I am staying at the right weight and finding the training is going so well. The advice just makes so much sense. My health is so important to me so I really like the idea of nourishing my body with only good foods."

"I'm so tired today from having stayed up to read your book last night. I couldn't put it down! It makes so much sense and I feel like you're standing here reading it to me when I'm going through it. It's like having a personal coach!"

"I need this book! The person who recommended it is literally fading away in front of my eyes but he's bouncing around with energy like Tigger – what has happened to him?!"

"Zoë, I am going to get there, thanks to you. I couldn't believe my eyes when I weighed this morning - I've lost a phenomenal 10lb already and this is only the beginning of Day 4! What's more, no hunger cravings whatsoever, and with the added benefit of my arthritic knees having stopped complaining. What joy to find a route back to a normal size - thanks once again for being caring and generous to share your findings and research."

"What an Easter present – both my partner and I have lost 10lb in 9 days – this is the fastest weight loss we have ever experienced – even more than on Atkins. What's more we feel great! We're sleeping well, the cravings have gone, we feel clear headed and just alive really. Thank you so much."

"Hi. Just thought I'd drop you a line to say that I am extremely impressed; I've lost half a stone since Friday and my trousers are falling down (could be a bit embarrassing really)! Here's to the next 6.5st! Thank you ever so much - the book is such an inspiration - my mum is going on it too."

"I'm doing brilliantly – 10lb in 2 weeks and 1 week of that was on holiday. I found it surprisingly easy to stick to on holiday – tropical fruits for breakfast one day and meat, cheese and omelette the next. The fat meals were dead easy for main meals and I just wasn't hungry. I even cheated with quite a lot of alcohol and I still lost weight."

"Hubby has lost 9lb now in 2 weeks – he hasn't even really been trying, sod him! And he hasn't even read the book – he just phones me up and says 'can I have this?' and I say 'yes' or 'no'. Men!"

"I read 4 pages and lost two and a half stone – I figured I'd better not read much more!"

CONTENTS

Foreword   xi

Part 1 – Introduction & Background   1

1   Good days and bad days: *What this book is all about*   2
2   ER: *The minimum medical jargon you need to understand*   15
    why you overeat

Part 2 – The Definition Of Madness   27

3   You may as well count stars: *Why calorie counting doesn't*   29
    work
4   "Pure White & Deadly": *Sugar – the more accessible heroin*   33
5   Eating fat doesn't make you fat: *Fat is not the enemy – let it*   38
    be your friend
6   Cabbage soup for the soul: *You need never try another fad*   49
    diet again

Part 3 – Why Do You Overeat?
When All You Want Is To Be Slim   51

7   Calorie counting makes you fat: *It doesn't make you slim it*   54
    actually makes you fat
8   "I'm Sam and I'm a food addict": *Food addiction and food*   57
    cravings
9   How your gut flora are making you fat: *Candida – everything*   60
    you need to know
10 One person's poison: *Food Intolerance – everything you*   75
    need to know
11 Blood glucose – too low or too high?: *Hypoglycaemia –*   87
    everything you need to know
12 Completing the jigsaw: *Candida, Food Intolerance and*   94
    Hypoglycaemia and how overeating links with all of them

Part 4 – Eating & Nutrition   103

13   Phase 1: *The 5 day kick-start eating plan*   111
14   Phase 2: *The weight loss eating plan*   122
15   Phase 3: *The life-long eating plan*   143
16   Keep taking the tablets: *Vitamins, Minerals and Nutrition*   155
17   Where's the sugar? *Food families & where to find hidden*   175
      ingredients

Part 5 – Rationalisation & Explanations   185

18   Does my bum look big in this?: *Why are more women than*   186
      men obese?
19   Fat bank accounts, slim progress: *Why has obesity got worse*   189
      as we have 'developed' as nations?
20   Once I start I can't stop: *Why do we get into vicious and*   192
      virtuous circles?

Part 6 – Psychological Factors   197

21   Eat to live or live to eat: *Why do we eat & why do we*   198
      overeat?
22   Fat is a humanist issue: *Eating disorders and the*   207
      psychological reasons for overeating
23   It's up to you!: *The most important chapter in this book*   212
      (once you are free from addiction)

Part 7 – Other Related Issues   227

24   "I'm Pat and I'm an Alcoholic": *How Candida, Food*   228
      Intolerance and Hypoglycaemia explain alcoholism
25   "Animals are my friends and I don't eat my friends": *Can*   231
      you follow this plan and still be vegetarian?
26   So can you bin the gym membership?: *Where does exercise*   233
      fit in with all of this?

Part 8 – Questions & Answers   237
80 frequently asked questions with straight talking answers

Part 9 – Positive Thinking   269
Motivational thoughts to change your eating for ever

Part 10 – Recipes   273
Quick & easy menus for all phases of the eating plan

FOREWORD

Why did I write this book?

This book has been many years in the making. I have notes as far back as 1980 and I have developed my views with over twenty years worth of research and experience. I was finally inspired to devote the time and energy to writing everything down by two television programmes. I saw them in the UK but I am sure they have been replicated in the US, if not started there first.

The first was called "*Inch Loss Island*" on a UK morning TV show and the second was called "*Fat Club.*" Inch Loss Island chose five people at the start of 2001 and took them off to an island where they received coaching from a doctor, nutritionist, life coach and fitness instructor. They had one week on the island receiving advice and coaching before they were sent back to the mainland to try to lose weight on their own. They were visited regularly by the 'experts' they met on the island and were also weighed at regular intervals.

Fat Club was remarkably similar except that the ten contestants were gathered together at a country home for a weekend and given access to a doctor, nutritionist, psychologist and fitness instructor. They then went home to apply their new found knowledge and returned one weekend a month for the next six months to chart their progress.

In both cases the people lost weight initially but, just a few months into the programme, people were barely losing weight or were actually even putting weight back on. An example guinea pig from Fat Club called Kelly started off at 245lb (she is 5ft 3in) and she lost 8lb the first month, 2 the next, 6 the next and then actually put on 2lb in the fourth month. The weight loss for the whole group of ten contestants was 104lb the first month and then just 18lb in the fourth month. At this fourth weigh-in one person had left the programme and three people had put on weight. Another person left the programme the following month. In Inch Loss Island the results were similar – they even started Inch Loss Island II a year later when the Inch Loss Island I hopefuls were still far from their goal weights.

There were two things that inspired me to write this book:
1) The despair that the overweight people showed when, despite trying so hard, their weight loss slowed or in some cases they started to put weight back on
2) The advice that they were given.

1) You would not be human if you did not want to reach out to those people – to feel their pain and to try to make their lives better in some way. The emotions were so raw and the tears so genuine that it would have taken a robot not to feel moved. The emotions were all the more touching in that 90% of the western world can empathise with their plight. If we are not on a diet now, we have been on one. If we are not overweight now, we have been or will be at some point in the future. One question just kept coming up again and again – those people want to lose weight so badly that they will humiliate themselves on national television to get access to people who may make them slim. They will wear swimsuits when they weigh 300lb and show their cellulite to the world, just for a chance to lose weight. Why, why, why do they overeat when all they want is to be slim?

2) The dietary advice for Inch Loss Island was as follows:
Breakfasts – All Bran, Special K, Fruit & Fibre, Cornflakes – all sugared breakfast cereals. The breakfasts suggested on the programme's web site have approximately 300 calories and 2-4g of fat.
Lunches – Many varieties of meat, fish or vegetable meals such as bacon, lettuce & tomato sandwich, crumpets, bagels, hot dogs, rice and pasta (little mention of whole-meal rice and pasta). The lunches suggested on the web site have approximately 400 calories and 2-14g of fat.
Dinners – Many varieties of meat, fish or vegetable meals, which included things like mash, chips/fries, pasta, rice and baked beans. The dinner menus on the web site have approximately 300-450 calories and 4-15g of fat.

The total daily allowance was, therefore, approximately 1000-1150 calories per day and could have as little as 8g of fat – depending on the meal options chosen. In essence the contestants were sold the calorie theory – if you eat fewer calories than you need you will lose weight. As you will see later on in this book, this will work – but only in the short term. I'm sure all of you reading this book have lost weight counting calories only to have put it back on and more.

The guinea pigs on the national TV shows were told to create a calorie deficit to lose weight i.e. to eat less than their bodies needed. The one difference, to previous pure calorie counting advice, was that they were advised not to eat a very low calorie diet but to reduce their calorie intake and to increase their level of exercise so that their calorie requirements increased. In other words – eat less than your body needs **and** increase your activity levels so that your body needs even more. Can you imagine a car mechanic giving such advice? Don't give your car the petrol it needs and then flog it even harder just to increase the need for fuel! It is laughable, but this is the advice that the desperate slimmers were given.

The nutritional advice included eating low fat foods, knowing how to spot high fat foods a mile away, but eating anything in moderation. How can you eat things that you crave in moderation? Why are smokers told to give up cigarettes totally rather than to have a few each day? Why are alcoholics told not to let one drink pass their mouth rather than to have a glass of wine now and again? Why on earth, therefore, are slimmers advised to eat the food, for which they have addict-like cravings, in moderation?!

Inevitably the slimmers struggled to lose weight, became obsessed with food, overate and felt terribly guilty when they did (how much worse a binge is when it is recorded as a failure on national TV). It was their plight that finally inspired me to pull the twenty years worth of notes together and write this book. The research I have done and the discoveries that I have made have changed my life. They can do the same for you.

Who am I?

Most of the diet books I have read have been written by doctors, or PhD students, who have given very technical descriptions of how the body works and what happens when we eat certain things. I have talked to many people, who want to lose weight, about diet books that they have read and almost all of them confessed that they skipped the medical jargon and just turned to the 'what do I eat?' section. They can get the gist of what the book is about (i.e. high carbohydrate/low fat or low carbohydrate/high fat) and they then see if it works.

I am not a doctor. I am just like you. I was anorexic at sixteen, bulimic by nineteen and I have fought food cravings to rival any drug addiction for many years. I have suffered all of the three conditions that I will share with you in this book. (I no longer suffer any of them and I know how to make sure that they never return). I had the great fortune to be treated by Dr Jonathan Brostoff whilst suffering one of them as a student at Cambridge University in England. I had a glucose tolerance test in hospital, for another of the three conditions, which was stopped as I passed out within an hour and a half of being given the glucose. I had the third condition diagnosed by a nutritionist over ten years ago. I have read every diet and healthy eating book under the sun and have spent years wondering why people overeat when all they want is to be slim.

Why do obese people we see in the streets 'let themselves get like that' we ask (as if they have chosen to be that size). When we lose weight and feel great why do we overeat and put it back on? Why do we overeat to the extent that we feel ill? Why do we overeat in a way that doesn't even let us savour and enjoy the food we are eating? Why does food rule our lives? Why do we have 'good' days and 'bad' days? Why can't we stop overeating once we start? Why do we overeat when all we want is to be slim? **Why do you overeat? – When all you want is to be slim.**

This book has the answers to all these questions and more. I have found a way out of the cycle of overeating and out of the binge/starve cycle that so many of us get into. I know that the reason I **used to** overeat is because I had cravings that had to be experienced to be believed (but then I'm sure most of you know what I'm talking about). I now understand where the cravings come from and how to overcome them. I know that only when I am free from cravings can I control and really enjoy my eating.

I weigh 8st, which is 112lb (I am 5ft 2in) and have been at this weight for over ten years. I enjoy eating in a way I could never have dreamt of. I am no longer afraid of, or out of control with, food. I eat chocolate and indulge in Haagen-Dazs ice cream when I want to. I eat the same portions as my husband, who is almost double my size. The most frequent comment that friends and colleagues ever make to me is "*how can you possibly eat so much and stay so slim?*" This book will tell you how.

Some diet books will promise that you can eat what you like, when you like and be the size you like and you know that is nonsense. This book has three eating phases – the first will set you on the road to being free from food addiction. In many cases, if not most, this can take fewer than five days. The second phase is followed for as long as you want to lose weight. You will have just three 'rules' about what you can and can't eat but you will not be limited in the amount you eat and you will not go hungry. I have thought a great deal about what makes an eating plan workable and practical so Phase 2 is intended to be followed easily by business executives, busy parents, students and anyone else keen to lose weight. In Phase 3 you really, honestly will be able to eat what you want **almost** when you want. You will know how to make sure that food cravings don't return, you will know how much you can have of what you want and how often and you may actually find that many of the foods you crave like an addict right now hold no interest for you in little more than five days.

I feel desperately sorry for every overweight person who is still trying to fight food cravings on a daily, sometimes hourly, basis when they would give anything to be slim. I want to share the way out with you. I want to help you answer the question – **Why do you overeat? – When all you want is to be slim.**

PART 1

INTRODUCTION & BACKGROUND

1

GOOD DAYS & BAD DAYS

What this book is all about

What is the problem?

As we started the new millennium, for the first time in human history, the number of overweight people rivalled the number of underweight people, according to a report from the Worldwatch Institute, a Washington, DC-based research organization. While the world's underfed population had declined slightly, since 1980, to 1.1 billion, the number of overweight people had surged to 1.1 billion.

The general measurement that is now used to define 'overweight' is called the Body Mass Index (BMI). This is a measure of body fat based on height and weight that applies to both men and women. It is calculated by taking a person's weight in kilograms and dividing this by their height in metres squared, e.g. a 70kg person with a height of 1.8m has a Body Mass Index (BMI) of 70/(1.8x1.8) = 21.6. This is in the normal range.

The guidelines are:
- A BMI of less than 18.5 is considered "Underweight"
- A BMI of 18.5 - 24.9 is considered "Normal"
- A BMI of 25 - 29.9 is considered "Overweight"
- A BMI of 30 or more is considered "Obese"

If you want some help calculating your own BMI there is a 'look up' table in Chapter 15 to help you. This works in inches and pounds if you don't do metric.

The slimming industry is a multi billion-dollar industry (estimated to be worth $33 billion in the US and £5 billion in the UK) and yet more than half of American adults are overweight (a BMI of over 25) and nearly a quarter are obese (a BMI of over 30). The UK is not far behind with current estimates that over half of British adults will be officially overweight within the next five years. It is a complete paradox – the more a nation seems to spend on slimming the more overweight its people are. It's the chicken and the egg question. Are the fattest nations trying to slim or is the attempt to slim making nations fat? The answer is actually both. It is a vicious circle – the more we try to eat less, the more we crave food, the more we overeat and the fatter we get. We then try even harder to eat less to correct this and the vicious circle spirals ever downwards. Vicious circles and virtuous circles are explained in more detail in Chapter 20. This book shows why trying to eat less, i.e. calorie counting, both directly and indirectly causes us to crave food and put on weight and it shows us how to break out of the vicious circle for ever.

Good days and bad days

There is a current epidemic of overeating. Millions of people in the developed world are waking each morning wondering whether the day will be 'good' or 'bad'. We are not thinking about the weather or about what we will do at work or leisure. We are thinking about what and how much we will eat.

On a 'good' day we will get through the time from when we get up to when we go to bed without overeating. The relevant words here are 'get through'. The day is never easy. Rather it is a constant battle of resistance, a continuous struggle against the urge to eat. Some people will go to great lengths to lessen the temptation – even to the extent of staying in bed or taking a trip into the countryside away from shops. In the UK, in the 1980s, there was a tragic story, which made national headlines, about a bulimic aerobics teacher who faked her own disappearance one December rather than face all the overeating opportunities that Christmas gives. How many of us empathised with her extreme measures. Any reader familiar with the 'good' day scenario will know that it ends with a sense of achievement but also an underlying fear that the period of being in control with food is likely to be short-lived. This is invariably the case.

On a 'bad' day we will not be able to resist the urge to eat and, having started, we may not be able to stop. Many overeaters eat so fast that they do not taste the food. Most rarely enjoy much more than the first mouthful, if that. Many eat way beyond the feeling of fullness. Many continue to eat even when they feel bloated or even physically sick. Yet we want more than anything else to be slim. Magazines ask which we would rather happen: to be and stay at our ideal weight for life; to win the lottery; to meet the partner of our dreams; or to land our dream job. Guess what comes top? How can we question the desire to be slim? It is at the top, heading the list, of the most desirable things in the world.

People are prepared to take tablets to slim or even contemplate stomach stapling or jaw wiring – how much does this tell you about their desire to be slim? And yet more of us than ever are overweight and the numbers are rising at an alarming rate. The one conclusion you have to reach is that what we are currently doing doesn't work. Counting calories, fad diets, slimming pills are clearly not the answer or obesity would not be an issue let alone an epidemic. Why, why, why, therefore, do we overeat?

Why do you overeat? – When all you want is to be slim

For too long the answer offered has been a psychological one – many overeaters are females and so the mother-daughter relationship has been seized upon by a host of post-Freudian writers. The issue of women's sexuality in the late twentieth/early twenty-first century has been discussed at length – the role of the supermodel and our magazine culture. Men are now also believed to be caught up in this magazine culture and under pressure to achieve a certain look. We are in the period of the greatest change known to humankind and the stress that this has caused has also been cited as a reason for our inability to follow a healthy eating plan. Many other suggestions have been made in an attempt to explain why, in developed societies, healthy food is more widely available than it has ever been and yet obesity and overeating are at record levels.

The psychological reasons behind overeating have a place in the theory of the condition but they are not sufficient as explanations. There is a lot going on psychologically when we overeat but far more important is what is going on physically. The willpower needed by overeaters to resist the urge to binge is so intense that it cannot be less than the desire an alcoholic has for a drink or a smoker has for a cigarette. Yet overeaters are treated as people with no willpower at best or a psychological condition at worst. Why are alcoholics and smokers treated as addicts with a physical problem (and possible secondary emotional problems) when overeaters are seen as people with a psychological disorder? Why are overeaters also not seen as addicts just like alcoholics or drug addicts?

The answer to the question that is the title of this book is that you overeat because you are in effect a food addict. Your cravings for food, which drive you to overeat, are as strong as those cravings experienced by drink or drug addicts. At the exact moment you overeat, your desire to eat is stronger than even your immense desire to be slim. You do desperately want to be slim. You wake up determined, you stick to a diet for a couple of hours or days but then you have a craving so overwhelming that you will drive to a 7-11 in the middle of the night or you will eat the children's sweets or you will possibly even take things out of the dustbin that you threw away yesterday to stop you eating them. You are not a failure. You are not greedy or weak willed. This is not your fault. You are addicted to food. You can, however, change this.

4

What is Food Addiction?

Addiction to a substance has four main characteristics:
1) An uncontrollable craving.
2) Increasing tolerance so that more of the addictive substance is needed in order to produce the same effects.
3) Physical or psychological dependence – the substance produces a feeling of well-being (euphoria in the extreme) when you first consume it and then, in the latter stages of the addiction, the substance is needed to avoid unpleasant withdrawal feelings.
4) Adverse effects on the consumer.

Food addicts will empathise with the above – let us look at the four characteristics of addiction in relation to chocolate as an example:
1) 'Chocoholics' will describe cravings for chocolate that are addict-like and quite uncontrollable.

2) The chocolate binges get worse and worse and 'chocoholics' feel the need to consume ever-increasing quantities of chocolate to satisfy their addiction.

3) The third characteristic – physical or psychological dependence – describes the situation where the addict stops getting good feelings when they eat chocolate. They actually get to the point where they need chocolate to stop the withdrawal symptoms, i.e. they need chocolate not to feel good but to stop feeling bad.

4) Finally, think about the adverse effects – the unbearable cravings, the dopey feelings, headaches, bloating, weight gain/fluctuations, water retention, fatigue and so on. If it were not for these you would have little reason to confront the problem – you would just carry on eating chocolate. But food addiction gets worse, not better and at some stage the adverse effects get so bad that you have to act.

In the above respects food addiction is exactly the same as alcoholism or drug addiction. Drug addicts get a fantastic high when they first take, say, heroin. Then, perhaps for a few occasions whilst taking the substance, they experience great highs. Very quickly, more quickly with some people than others, the highs wear off and the drug is then needed not to get high but to avoid the equal and opposite low, which becomes more and more unbearable. The craving for heroin becomes insatiable and more and more of the substance is needed to continually avoid the terror of the withdrawal symptoms. The adverse effects on the consumer at this stage are dreadful – tracks on the arms, tremors, sweats, severe weight loss, no energy, no life let alone zest for life, pale skin, shattered immune system, infections and possibly even HIV if needles have been shared. Food addiction differs from drug addiction only in the extreme lengths people will go to for their fix and perhaps in the strength of the adverse effects. In general, drug addiction leads to more physical and mental damage than food addiction. However, if you have seen a 200-300lb person with no energy or health or desire for life, existing day to day rather than living, you may wonder that there is little difference in the effect that food or heroin can have on our well-being.

Food addiction is absolutely devastating – it leads to the good and bad days described above. It can lead to the addict thinking of nothing but food from the minute that they wake until the minute that they go to bed, with every day being a battle of wills – fighting what you want to eat with what you think you should eat. Some days you win the fight, some days you don't.

To be a food addict means to no longer have control over your food consumption. Depending on the degree of your addiction it can also mean some, or all, of the following:

- To be obsessed with, yet terrified of, food.
- To think about food from the minute you wake up until the minute you fall asleep.
- To be terrified of putting on weight.
- To fear social situations where you may not be able to determine what food may be on offer.
- To decline social invitations for this reason.
- To decline social invitations because you want to lose weight before seeing so-and-so again.
- To judge a day purely by the amount of food you have, or have not, consumed, not by what you have done or achieved.
- To be overwhelmed with guilt for eating an apple if you vowed not to eat an apple that day.
- To hate yourself.
- To feel a failure.
- To decline a dinner invitation as you don't intend to eat that day.
- To decline a dinner invitation for the above reason and then stuff yourself for the entire evening instead.
- To make a fresh start each and every day.
- To be utterly demoralised by continuous failure.
- To lose all faith and confidence in yourself.
- To feel that you are having a nightmare that will never end.
- To waste vast amounts of potential because all your energy and ambition is being channelled into eating or not eating.

- To be unable to sleep some nights due to genuine hunger.
- To collapse into a heavy sleep after a binge and to wake the next morning puffy eyed, bloated, hungover and fat.
- To have two wardrobes.
- To be unable to plan ahead because you don't know what weight you will be and hence you won't know if you will even want to attend a social occasion, let alone what you will wear.
- To continually set yourself tougher and tougher 'rules' in an attempt to control your behaviour.
- To feel totally out of control nonetheless.
- To hate the lies and deception which accompany food addiction as you try to avoid food or social occasions.
- To want to be open but to feel the world will despise you.
- To put off living until tomorrow *"when I'll be slim."*
- To exist not to live!

If you empathise with any, or all, of the above statements this book is for you. The above list describes a nightmare – the most horrible place to be. I wrote the above list back in the 1980s when my eating was out of control. I read the list now and struggle to empathise with it at all but I am so glad that I kept the notes I wrote then to remind me of a place I never want to return to. To be a healthy, slim person living inside a fat body is literally to feel that you cannot live with yourself. You want to escape your body and leave the fat that you loathe so much behind. The pain and despair faced by food addicts knows no limits. But there is a way out. There is a way to stop the food addiction and to stop the overeating. This is what this book is about.

However, saying that we overeat because we are food addicts is a bit of a tautology – it is just saying the same thing in a different way. It would be like saying we are alcoholics because we crave alcohol. Or, we are drug addicts because we crave drugs. So what we really need to answer, to get to the crux of the issue is – why are we food addicts? Why do we overeat? **Why do you overeat? – When all you want is to be slim.**

Why are you a food addict?

There are psychological reasons which lead people to become dependent on food. Food does act as a comfort, a stress release, an escape. Food is like alcohol to many overeaters – when we binge we are so 'spaced out' we may as well be drunk – this may be our way of coping with the world. We do need to be aware of, and deal with, any psychological factors that may be playing a part in our overeating.

However, much stronger than this, there are physical reasons why we overeat.

You overeat and binge compulsively because of one thing that you are doing and because of one, or all, of three conditions which you may have. The one thing that you are doing is calorie counting (by this I mean trying to eat fewer calories than your body needs) and this book will show how this leads directly to overeating by itself. There are then three conditions that you may have, which lead to immense food cravings, and these are Candida, Food Intolerance and Hypoglycaemia. You will also see how calorie counting contributes to Candida, Food Intolerance and Hypoglycaemia so you will see how calorie counting both directly and indirectly leads to food addiction. You may have one, or all, of these conditions and any, or all, of them will lead to addict-like cravings. You are not weak willed. You are not greedy. You have a health problem, or a number of health problems, and you must think of yourself as similar to a diabetic in that there are certain foods that you simply must avoid for your health. You are an alcoholic with food in place of alcohol. You are a nicotine addict with food in place of cigarettes.

Having compared food addiction to drink or drug addiction, there is a key factor which makes the treatment of an eating problem far more difficult than that of a drink or drug addiction. The problem is this – an alcoholic is advised to go 'cold turkey' (to totally avoid drink) just as a smoker has to totally avoid cigarettes. Indeed reformed alcoholics stick tightly to the principle 'one day at a time' and they think just one taste of alcohol could set them back on the downhill path to alcoholism. The problem for the food addict is that they cannot go 'cold turkey' (excuse the pun) on food. Overeaters have to eat but not binge. That is like telling a drug addict to have some heroin each day but not too much! A sure recipe for disaster.

Many overeaters would agree that it is easier to ban food totally than it is to eat it in moderation. The continued success of liquid diets since the 1980s supports this – many overeaters find it easier to survive on fewer than 500 calories a day, all in liquid form, than to eat real food in a calorie counted diet.

The current advice on overeating seems to be to eat everything in moderation. Many slimming clubs tell us we can eat anything, but we have to count the points allocated to each food (another way of counting calories). With calorie counting, we are told we can eat anything so long as we don't exceed a certain number of calories a day. We are told that no food is a sin, no food is bad for us and if we ban foods we will simply crave them. Why don't we advise the alcoholic to have a glass of wine and a measure of spirits but not a whole bottle of either? Why don't we say to the smoker don't give up cigarettes or you will only crave them? This advice would be simply crazy for drink or drug addicts so how, therefore, can it possibly work for the overeater?

The fundamental problem is that food addiction is not seen as a similar problem to any other addiction. It is widely accepted that drugs, alcohol and cigarettes are addictive but it is less widely accepted that food can be addictive (although caffeine is being increasingly recognised as an addictive substance). However, in many ways, your problem is worse. An alcoholic can overcome their problem by avoiding alcohol altogether. A nicotine addict must give up cigarettes. A drug addict must stop taking drugs. You, a food addict, cannot stop eating. You have to learn to live with food and to eat in such a way that you don't overeat and, most importantly, that you don't have an uncontrollable desire to overeat. Fortunately, there is a way to do this...

What is the way out?

1) The first thing that you have to do is to stop calorie counting. Before you panic and throw this book away, ask yourself why you are reading it. Has calorie counting worked for you? Have you lost weight and kept it off? Are you at your ideal weight and are you free from food cravings? No!

Please read Chapter 3 and Chapter 7 on calorie counting before you try to hang on to this 'comfort blanket' any longer. Calorie counting has got you into the mess you're in now and stopping it is the only way out. Not only does calorie counting not work, it leads directly and indirectly to food cravings, which is the reason why you overeat. You have to stop counting calories if you want to lose weight. Have faith, dare to try something different and please keep reading.

2) The second thing that you have to do is to understand which of the three conditions you are suffering from, identify the foods that contribute to these conditions and stop eating these foods. You don't go 'cold turkey' on food but you do go 'cold turkey' on the foods that are contributing to your addict-like cravings. There are bad foods. Some food is good for you and some is not and you have to start nourishing your body, not stuffing and starving it. You also have to stop trying to be an addict in moderation! You are trying to stop being a smoker by having a few a day. You are trying to stop being an alcoholic by having a couple of glasses a day. Eating what you crave in moderation really is that crazy. The sooner you stop trying to (quite literally) have your cake and eat it, the sooner you will free yourself from cravings and be able to control your eating.

Who is this book for?

This book is for anyone who wants to lose weight. It is especially for those who want to lose weight so desperately that they can't think what they would like more than this. It is for anyone who has ever calorie counted, lost weight, put weight back on or put more back on than they first lost! It is for anyone who has food cravings or feels that they are addicted to food in some way. It is for anyone who will go out of their way, day or night, to get the food that they are craving. In short this book is for you, if you can't understand why you overeat when all you want is to be slim.

How can this book help?

By telling you the one thing that you are doing to virtually guarantee you will overeat.
By telling you the three key physical reasons for your overeating.
By helping you identify which of these may be issues for you and how you overcome them.
By explaining how calorie counting has got you to where you are today.
By giving you the chance to eat to live rather than living to eat.
By giving you a life-long eating plan which will help you:

- Lose weight and keep the weight off,
- Overcome cravings for good,
- Gain energy and better health,
- Stop starving and bingeing,
- Get on with your life rather than calorie counting all day long.

You are not weak willed. It is not your fault that you are overweight or that you overeat. You are up against some physical cravings that are quite overwhelming. Take the first step to fighting them and read this book. It will help you achieve all of the above and more. More energy, better health and a life free from food addiction.

What is this book saying?

This book argues that food addiction is a very real problem and that the epidemic of overeating should be treated as a physical, not just a psychological, condition. The growing number of eating disorders and the increased incidence of obesity should be viewed as a physical issue. Its prevalence in the late twentieth century and now the twenty-first century can be explained by conditions such as Candida, Food

Intolerance and Hypoglycaemia. Each of these can lead to intolerable food cravings and food addiction.

Whole chapters, in this book, are devoted to Candida, Food Intolerance and Hypoglycaemia. What are they? How do they develop in a person? What effect do they have? What are the symptoms and how can the conditions be overcome? The key issue of interest in this book, however, is how they contribute to overeating and intolerable food cravings, because all of them do.

What if you are not weak willed but instead a food addict with cravings for certain foods that all the willpower in the world wouldn't be able to overcome? If someone would go so far as to have surgery to lose weight, should we question their desire to be slim? No – it is paramount! What if Candida, Food Intolerance and Hypoglycaemia are driving you to consume specific foods in excessive quantities, when these are the very foods and quantities that wreck your diet? What if there was a way to channel the willpower you undoubtedly do have into a more productive battle that can help you win the slimming war?

The essence of this book is that you will continue to overeat, to crave food uncontrollably, unless you identify and avoid all foods to which you are addicted. Cravings will be out of your control for as long as you have Candida, Food Intolerance and/or Hypoglycaemia, which are out of control. Take Candida as an example. We will see later in this book that Candida is a parasite, which can become widespread in our bodies and it thrives on foods like yeast and sugar. Consequently rampant Candida in your body will cry out for anything which contains these substances – hence the cravings you may have for bread, cereal, sweets, chocolate, ice cream etc. With Food Intolerance, the real paradox here is that your body is most likely to crave the very substance(s) to which you are intolerant. Hence again, a physical condition can generate intense and specific food cravings. Finally, Hypoglycaemia will result in a lowering of your body's blood glucose level, which again will make your body cry out for sugary substances.

PART 1 will introduce some medical terms in the simplest possible language. To understand how to lose weight we need to understand things like:
- How does the body turn food into energy?
- Or, perhaps more importantly, how does the body turn food into fat?
- Why is insulin called the fattening hormone?

We will keep the jargon to the minimum but there are some medical terms that will really help you understand why you overeat and why you are overweight.

PART 2 will challenge what you may believe at the moment. You have probably been on every fad diet under the sun – all of which control calories in some way or another. The definition of madness was once explained to me as doing the same thing over and over again and expecting a different result. You have tried all the diets around to date and failed. Therefore, you have to try something different. You have to have the courage to throw out some of the things you have held to be true for so long:

- **Counting calories doesn't work** – You have to stop counting calories and start nurturing your body. Don't stop reading now. You won't put on weight. Keep reading and you will discover how to lose weight and then maintain your weight without counting calories. It is **what** you eat not **how much** that is important.
- **Sugar is the enemy** – You may have been told that fat is the enemy. Cut out fat and lose weight. When food manufacturers cut fat they need to put something back in to compensate for the taste loss – this is invariably sugar in one form or another. Sugar is messing up your body mechanisms and your weight loss attempts in the process.
- **Fat is not the enemy** – fat is tasty and necessary for our health and you are cutting it out unnecessarily. There are different types of fat, however, and some are good for you and some aren't.
- **Fad diets don't work** – you must know this makes sense, so hopefully this chapter will be preaching to the converted.

PART 3 will really get to the crux of the issue – **Why do you overeat? – When all you want is to be slim**. Read it and see. We will explore some things that you have probably heard of like Candida, Food Intolerance and Hypoglycaemia and show how they all fit together and all explain the many health problems you may have been experiencing.

- What is Candida? What is Food Intolerance? What is Hypoglycaemia?
- What are the links between Candida, Food Intolerance and Hypoglycaemia?
- How does overeating link in with all of them?
- What are the symptoms? How are they caused? How can they be controlled?
- What is addiction? How does it relate to Candida, Food Intolerance and Hypoglycaemia?

PART 4 will cover diet & nutrition:

- Which diets are recommended for people suffering from Candida, Food Intolerance and Hypoglycaemia?
- Is there a 'perfect' diet?

- What about vitamins, minerals & nutrition?
- How will you feel short, medium and long term if you change your eating habits?
- How can you never go hungry again?
- How can you eat to live, not live to eat?

PART 5 will show how the rationale in this book explains other things that you may have noticed:
- Why are more women than men obese?
- Why has obesity got progressively worse as we have 'developed' as nations?
- Why do we get into vicious and virtuous circles?

PART 6 looks at the psychological aspects of overeating:
- Why do we eat? Why do we overeat?
- What are eating disorders?
- What does it mean to be a food addict?
- How can you change your frame of mind so that you can be more in control of food?
- What are the two voices going on in your head telling you to be 'good' one minute and then 'bad' the next?
- When you are free from food addiction and can make a real choice about what you eat – what will you choose?

PART 7 will come onto other related issues:
- Does food addiction have anything to say about alcoholism? Is there a way in which the eating plan to overcome Candida, Food Intolerance and Hypoglycaemia can also help alcoholics with their addiction?
- Where does vegetarianism fit in? Can you follow this book's advice and still be vegetarian? (The short answer is yes, because I'm a vegetarian).
- Do you need to exercise?

PART 8 is a straight talking Question & Answer section. There are 80 direct questions with no nonsense answers. Fundamentally, this book will answer the question – **Why do you overeat? – When all you want is to be slim.** It will also answer many more such as – Why have you failed so many times before? Why will you succeed this time?

PART 9 concludes this book with positive thinking and personal motivation tips to provide inspiration as you set off on your life changing journey.

PART 10 has some recipes that you may enjoy. They are clearly labelled so that you can see which are suitable for vegetarians and different phases of the eating plan.

A small request...

Please read this book all the way through, in the right order, before leaping into a new way of eating. It will be so tempting to jump to the section on 'what you can eat' just to see if you can stick to it. If you need to do that, please do it now and then come back to the beginning and read everything all the way through. You are going to be asked to throw away some beliefs that you may have held onto for some time and to try some new things and you really need to understand **why**, before you will agree to do this. This book tells you how, why, when, what, who, all the way through, so please let it help you on your journey – thank you.

KEY POINTS FROM CHAPTER 1

- Our desire to be slim is unquestionable – there must be something even more powerful going on to stop us achieving this goal. There is! The 'more powerful thing' is food cravings.
- Whilst psychological reasons for overeating are important to understand, there are physical reasons that are just as important, if not more so.
- We overeat because we are food addicts, with addict-like cravings.
- We have addict-like cravings because of calorie counting (which makes us crave any food) and because of Candida, Food Intolerance and/or Hypoglycaemia (which make us crave specific foods).
- The only route to stopping overeating is to stop the cravings.
- Food addiction should be taken as seriously as alcoholism and drug/cigarette addiction. No one would tell an alcoholic or drug addict to drink or inject in moderation! To give such advice to food addicts is equally ludicrous.
- Calorie counting doesn't work – worse still it actually makes you fat.

2

EMERGENCY ROOM (ER)

**The minimum medical jargon you need
to understand why you overeat**

Most of the books I have read on diets, healthy eating, nutrition, Candida, Food Intolerance and Hypoglycaemia have been written by doctors and there are many pages of medical references, which I have skipped over as things such as prostaglandins, immunoglobulins and phagocytic cells have not interested me. All I wanted to know was how I could get into my jeans by Saturday! If your reaction to medical jargon is the same I will try to explain some terms that we do need to understand as simply as possible. Please do persevere with this section as it really is useful to understand how your body uses the food that you eat and what, therefore, is causing your fat. If we can answer the following...
- How does the body turn food into energy?
- And more importantly how does it turn food into fat?
- What is insulin?
- Why is insulin called the fattening hormone?
- What happens if blood glucose is high?
- Why is diabetes so lethal?
...we can understand the keys to weight loss much better.

What do we eat?

All the food that we eat is one, or more, of the following:
- Carbohydrate
- Fat
- Protein

This is worth repeating. Everything we eat is a carbohydrate, a fat or a protein or a combination of two, or all three, of these.

Carbohydrates are the substances that are most easily converted into glucose (fuel) to supply energy to the body. They can be categorised in many different ways. However, the only categorisation that we are interested in is refined carbohydrates vs. **un**refined carbohydrates.

Understanding the difference between these is one of the key weapons in the war against overeating.

- Refined carbohydrates are carbohydrates that have been altered in some way from their natural form. e.g. apple juice is refined because apple juice doesn't grow on trees. Chips are refined because they don't come out of the ground.
- Unrefined carbohydrates are carbohydrates that are eaten as they would be found in their natural form. Whole eating apples are unrefined because they do grow on trees in that exact form. Potatoes in their jackets are unrefined because they do come out of the ground in that exact form.

Fats are crucial for our well-being as they form the membrane (thin protection layer) that surrounds every cell in our bodies. With the right fats our cells are strong, without them they are weak and prone to attack. The right fats give us Essential Fatty Acids which are crucial for our optimal health.

Fat comes from two sources:
1) Animal sources – meat, fish, cheese, eggs and dairy foods – these are generally solid at room temperature.
2) Vegetable sources – peanut oil, olive oil, sunflower oil – these are generally liquid at room temperature.

We can also categorise fat as saturated fat, monounsaturated fat, polyunsaturated fat and transunsaturated fat (also known as hydrogenated fat). We will learn more about fat in Chapter 5.

The word **Protein** comes from a Greek word meaning basic or fundamental. Proteins are essential parts of all living things so we need to eat protein to keep all parts of our body healthy – muscles, organs, the brain and our bones.

Protein comes from two sources:
1) Animal sources – meat, fish, cheese, eggs and dairy foods.
2) Vegetable sources – nuts, whole grains, beans, pulses and tofu.

Which foods are Protein or Carbohydrate or Fat?

Pure protein and fat has no carbohydrate at all. Meat and fish for example have protein and fat in differing proportions, depending on how lean or fatty they are, but they have no carbohydrate. Butter is almost entirely fat. It has a trace of protein but no carbohydrate. Most other foods have traces of all three – carbohydrate, fat and protein – but they fit into one main category. Fruits, for example, have traces of protein and fat but essentially they are carbohydrates. Some foods do have a high amount of more than one category – for example beans and pulses are both protein and carbohydrate, meat and fish are both protein and fat. Real milk is one of the rare products that is all three in good measure – a carbohydrate, a fat and a protein. Maybe this is why it is such a complete food for infants. Nuts also have significant amounts of carbohydrate, fat and protein. Below is a diagram to show which foods fit into mainly one category and which fit into more than one or even all three categories:

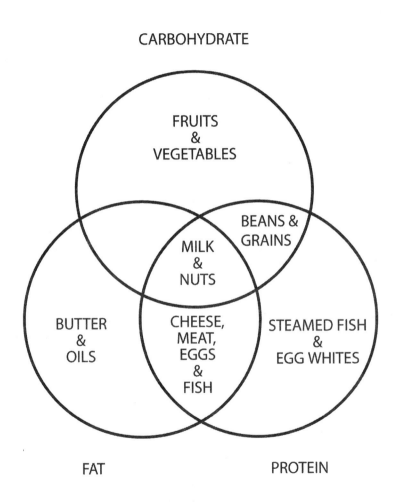

This diagram has real importance for the rationale of the eating plan in this book. We will come onto this in detail in Part 4 on Eating & Nutrition. The key things we need to remember from the previous diagram are:

- Meat, fish, cheese and eggs are essentially fat. Fruits, vegetables and grains (rice, wheat, barley etc) are essentially carbohydrates. The two groups should not be eaten at the same time. Lots more on this later.
- Milk and nuts, foods which have carbohydrate, fat and protein in substantial quantities, should be eaten with care. We explain why later.
- There are some foods that are so low in carbohydrate, fat and protein that they can be eaten freely, at any time, with any meals or in between meals. These are generally green foods or 'rabbit food' as we sometimes call them. They include lettuce, salad leaves, cucumber, celery and green cabbage leaves as the key examples. They are essentially water so we don't have to worry about how much, or when, we eat these.

What are the other bits we need to know about?

We need to know about the 'sugar' handling parts of the body. We need to know about the level of glucose in the blood and how it changes. The term 'blood sugar' is often used when talking about blood glucose. However, I will only use the term blood glucose when talking about the level of glucose found in our blood to avoid confusion with the sugar we eat (the sugar that we put in drinks or eat in confectionery bars etc). This 'table' sugar does have an effect on our blood glucose level but we need to keep the sugar we eat separate from what happens to our blood glucose level to avoid confusion.

Our normal levels of blood glucose are around 65 to 110mg per 100cc of blood. When our blood glucose level stays above this the impact is serious and can even be fatal. Without knowing the medical detail of high, low and normal blood glucose levels you will probably be familiar with the effects. When you eat a confectionery bar, biscuit, cake or something similar, you may experience a surge of energy as the glucose floods into your blood stream – literally a sugar high. Low blood glucose is what you may have experienced, often late morning, late afternoon, or soon after a sugar high, when you feel irritable, hungry, have difficulty concentrating and may even have slightly shaky hands. The body's blood glucose level is crucial to our well-being and it is also crucial to our desire to lose weight.

The things we need to know about the body and sugar handling are:

The **Pancreas** is an organ in the body located below and behind the stomach. Its main functions are a) to produce the hormones insulin and glucagon and b) to produce digestive enzymes to help digest (break down) the food that we eat. The pancreas is a key organ in the digestion of food and the maintenance of our blood glucose level. When the pancreas doesn't work the person is defined as diabetic (full definition below).

Insulin is a hormone produced by the pancreas. When we eat a carbohydrate our body converts this into glucose and so the level of glucose in our blood rises. This is dangerous for the human body so we have this fantastic mechanism within the pancreas which ensures that insulin is released from the pancreas to 'mop up' the excess glucose and to return our blood glucose level to normal.

Glucagon is another hormone produced by the pancreas. Glucagon helps insulin keep our blood glucose level in the normal range. Not to be confused with…

Glycogen is a large molecule (starch) made up of glucose units. It is an energy store. Most of it is held in the liver and the muscle cells and there is generally less than 1kg , 2lb, of it in the body.

Glucose is the primary fuel used by most cells in the body to generate the energy that is needed to carry out their functions. (It is the petrol in our engines in effect).

Diabetes literally means "*sweet urine.*" It is a medical condition, which has been known to doctors for thousands of years. (References to this disease can be found in many ancient writings). In people who have diabetes the pancreas does not work properly. In this situation, when diabetics eat, their blood glucose level rises but the pancreas does not release enough, or any, insulin to return the blood glucose level to normal. The fact that sugar is passed through the body and found in the urine is the cast iron test for the presence of diabetes.

There are two types of diabetes:
- Type I diabetes is called "*Juvenile diabetes*" and is generally very sudden and serious and affects young people commonly around the ages of ten to twelve. People experience a sudden and dramatic weight loss, insatiable thirst and the situation can be fatal if they are not diagnosed and treated very quickly.

- Type II diabetes is called "*Maturity onset diabetes*" and can affect people of any age and is often found in overweight people. It can also affect pregnant women when their blood glucose level is affected by their pregnancy.

Type I diabetes almost always needs to be treated with insulin injections whereas Type II diabetes can more often be controlled by diet. The vast majority of diabetics, 95%, have Type II diabetes. The causes of both types of diabetes are not exactly known but risk factors (things that increase your chance of getting diabetes) include: having a family history of diabetes; being obese or overweight; physical inactivity; older age and race/ethnicity. People with a family history of diabetes are more likely to develop the condition themselves. Overweight people are more likely than normal weight people to become diabetic. People who don't take exercise are more at risk. The risk increases the older you get so older people are more likely to get Type II diabetes. Finally, African Americans and Hispanic/Latino Americans are twice as likely to get diabetes as Caucasians although we don't know exactly why.

The International Diabetes Federation (IDF) states that there were 194 million people with diabetes world wide in 2003. They estimate that there will be 333 million by 2025. The US has 15.3 million diabetics, which is over 6% of the US population. Only India and China have higher numbers of diabetics and this is due to the size of their populations. They have 32.7 million and 22.6 million respectively. Diabetes is the third leading cause of death in the US after heart disease and cancer. It is the leading cause of blindness and sight defects in developed countries and is the leading cause of amputations where an accident has not happened.

5.7% of the European population has diabetes, 32 million adults. Of these 1.6 million have Type I Diabetes and the other 30.4 million have Type II. (www.idf.org)

What happens when we eat?

When you eat something, your body absorbs certain substances from your food, mostly across the surface of your small intestine. As this happens, food is literally entering your body for use.

From the carbohydrates you eat, your body will absorb simple sugars, all of which either are, or quickly and easily become, glucose. From fat the body absorbs fatty acids and from protein it absorbs amino acids, the building blocks of protein. Although we can make energy from all three types of food – carbohydrate, fat and protein – carbohydrates are the easiest foods from which to get fuel. Our bodies need the simplest form of carbohydrate as fuel – glucose – and, therefore, the body turns carbohydrates into glucose as the first step to giving us fuel. (As we will see in Chapter 16 on vitamins and minerals – we need more than just carbohydrates for energy. We also need eight vitamins and five minerals for the enzymes in our body to drive the energy burner. The eight vitamins needed are the B family – B1, B2, B3, B5, B6, B12, folic acid and biotin. The minerals needed are iron, calcium, magnesium, chromium and zinc).

When we eat carbohydrates our body decides how much of the energy taken in is needed immediately and how much should be stored for future requirements. As our blood glucose level rises, insulin is released from the pancreas and this insulin converts some of the glucose to glycogen, a starch stored in the muscles and the liver available for energy use. Glycogen is our energy store room, if you remember from the definitions above. The next bit is the most important bit of all to remember: **If all the glycogen storage areas are full, insulin will convert the excess to fatty tissue. This is why insulin has been called the fattening hormone.**

Why do we need to know all this?

We need to know these basics because the hormone insulin is of real importance in our overeating and desire to lose weight. Insulin is the fattening hormone and the amount of insulin released into the body has a huge impact on our weight levels. Think about the following:
- Do you know anyone who has suddenly developed Type I diabetes? When juvenile diabetics first develop the disease, their pancreas literally stops working overnight and no insulin is produced. It is quite common for juvenile diabetics to lose 10lb or more in days as the production of insulin literally stops overnight. What does that tell us about insulin and weight loss?
- Then, when diabetics start injecting insulin on a daily basis, many struggle with their weight and many diabetics remain overweight for a lifetime. Again – what does that tell us about insulin and weight loss?
- High fat/protein, zero carbohydrate diets do have a dramatic impact on weight loss. This is because a diet with no carbohydrates in effect stops the production of insulin. Pure fat and protein (meat, fish and dairy products for example) do not cause the pancreas to release insulin. If you eat nothing but fat and protein, for even a short period of time, despite the fact that your calorie intake may be high, you will see a rapid weight loss. (I am not recommending this as a balanced diet but it does tell us how to harness this information for use in a more balanced weight loss approach).

Just think about these facts again – your body stops producing insulin and you lose weight more dramatically than with any other illness. You start taking insulin in injections and your weight goes back up. You stop insulin production by not eating carbohydrates and your weight falls. These facts alone are convincing that insulin is an incredibly powerful hormone and an important issue in weight loss.

We don't know everything we need to know about insulin but we do know that it acts to control the level of glucose in the body. We also know that it facilitates the storage of fat. **As only carbohydrates trigger the release of insulin, the secret to weight loss lies with carbohydrates.** If you restrict carbohydrate intake, you reduce the production of insulin, which is the hormone that facilitates the storage of fat.

If you look up any of the above terms – insulin, pancreas, glucose, glycagon, diabetes – on the Internet, or in encyclopaedias, you will be stunned by the complexity of the workings of just this part of the human body, let alone the whole thing. You may have two reactions:

1) Complete awe at the marvel that is a human being.
2) Complete horror at what we do to these incredibly sophisticated and sensitive mechanisms in our bodies on a daily, if not hourly, basis.

The human body is the true wonder of the world. We have over 200 bones and all the muscles and ligaments needed to move this complex structure with suppleness, stamina and strength. Some of us can run 100 metres in fewer than 10 seconds. Others can walk across the globe in months. Our heart is one of the most reliable pumps on earth. It will beat approximately 70 times a minute, 60 minutes an hour, 24 hours a day, 365 days a year for over 70 years. How awesome is that? Our bodies repair themselves and fight infection. They digest food efficiently and manage their own waste production. We can fly to the moon, cause, or prevent, other species becoming extinct, laugh, cry or tap dance! We are truly remarkable. Perhaps the most remarkable feature of the human being, however, is that we can do all of this despite the 'junk' that many of us put into our bodies. In this magnificent human body there is a mechanism which is trying to maintain a blood glucose level of around 65 to 110mg per 100cc of blood. How the body does this at all, let alone given what we eat, is just amazing.

Our pancreas was not designed to cope with mass produced modern foods. We started out eating animals, fruits, berries and things that we could find in the environment around us. These foods had negligible impact on our blood glucose level and, therefore, placed little strain on our pancreas and insulin production. We did not start out eating confectionery, chips and burgers with additives, preservatives, sugars and whatever else the modern manufacturing process has conjured up. No wonder then that our bodies are literally breaking down trying to cope with the junk that we put in them. We wouldn't try to run our car on the kind of rubbish we put into our own bodies. Putting diesel in a petrol car will grind it to a halt pretty quickly. We do much worse than this, to our far more sophisticated bodies on a daily, if not hourly, basis.

The pancreas is there to help us digest food and to ensure that our blood glucose level remains stable. Without the hormone insulin, which the pancreas produces, we would die. It is as simple as that. The pancreas detects what a person has eaten and releases the appropriate amount of insulin to maintain a healthy blood glucose level. When we eat in the way our ancestors did, the mechanism works well. When we eat meat, fish and plain vegetables our body releases hardly any insulin and our blood glucose level remains stable. When we drink a carton of apple juice our pancreas thinks we have eaten, say, twenty apples and releases the appropriate amount of insulin for twenty apples. When we eat a confectionery bar I dread to think what the pancreas thinks it is trying to cope with. What we do know is that the pancreas releases a significant amount of insulin to cope with the sugar onslaught. When we eat anything other than the whole food (apple juice instead of an apple, sugar instead of sugar cane, white rice instead of the whole grain) our bodies pump out too much insulin. This then lowers our blood glucose to below the level it was before we ate the food. This is essential to understand as it plays a huge part in food cravings and quite literally defines Hypoglycaemia, which is one of the cornerstones of this book.

Blood Glucose Levels

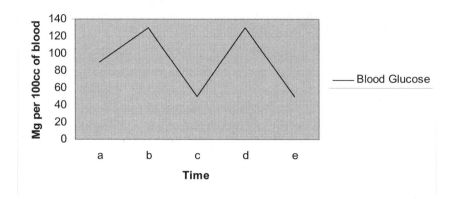

a) In the diagram above, at position 'a' your blood glucose level is stable at approximately 90mg per 100cc of blood.

b) You then eat a confectionery bar and at position 'b' your blood glucose level rises instantly (this is the sugar high/energy high that you experience).

c) Your pancreas then releases insulin to cope with the many pieces of fruit or equivalent sweetness that it thinks you have just eaten and at position 'c' your blood glucose level drops below where it was before you ate the confectionery bar.

d) This is when your body cries out to be fed and, if you reach for more confectionery, your blood glucose level will shoot back up again as at position 'd'.

e) More insulin will be released and your blood glucose level will then fall below normal levels again, as shown at position 'e', as too much insulin has been released to cope with the second confectionery bar.

When your blood glucose level drops below approximately 65mg per 100cc of blood, your cravings for food will be huge as your body is literally in danger mode. Your blood glucose has dropped to a level which is detrimental to your health and your body will try to do anything to get you to eat to raise your blood glucose level back to normal. If you have a banana or a similar whole carbohydrate you have a good chance of stabilising your blood glucose level. However, if you reach for another confectionery bar you will start the cycle all over again.

This is why once you start eating sweet foods (sweets, ice cream, chocolate, biscuits, cakes etc) you can't stop. It is so much easier not to have chocolate at all than it is to try to eat a limited amount – this really is like asking an alcoholic to have one drink and no more!

This is also why you may find it easier to eat nothing, rather than to try to eat a small amount. When you 'starve' (don't eat) your blood glucose level is low but at least it is stable. Hence, cravings are actually easier to control when you eat nothing!

Anything else I should know?

Yes! There are two other things that you should be aware of if you continue to stress your pancreas and insulin production unreasonably:
1) You will become more susceptible to diabetes – maturity onset diabetes generally.
2) There is a condition called *Syndrome X*, also called 'insulin resistance', which has become big in health news quite recently. *Syndrome X* is the phrase used to describe people who are identified as more susceptible to the workings of the pancreas and insulin production. Their bodies are described as 'insulin resistant' which means that their bodies are unresponsive to the release of insulin. With insulin resistance, eating refined carbohydrates causes lots of insulin to be released but the body fails to utilise this insulin efficiently and, therefore, the carbohydrates get stored as more fat instead, thus adding to your weight problem further. Tests have been developed to help identify people in the early stages of *Syndrome X* who are showing signs of insulin resistance and for whom diabetes and heart disease are likely to be problems later in life. It has been shown that 92% of people with Type II diabetes have insulin resistance. It is hoped that, by identifying the signs as early as possible, people may be able to change their eating patterns to avoid serious health problems in the future.

What is the relevance of all this in this book?

This book can be viewed as a jigsaw puzzle. You have probably heard about some, or all, of the key pieces in the jigsaw – calorie counting, Candida, Food Intolerance, Hypoglycaemia, insulin, sugar, fat etc. – this book will piece all of them together and show you that there is one consistent explanation for everything you have read. You may have read one book and thought one thing and then read another and thought you needed to try something different. You have probably read so many diet books you don't know what to believe and which way to turn. This book makes sense of the others and pieces together the jigsaw for you to make the one compelling message – the way forward to the new slim you. Chapter 12 will pull everything together with one diagram showing the causes and outcomes of everything related to food cravings and overeating.

What else can I read if I want to know more?

"Beat Stress & Fatigue" by Patrick Holford (1999)
"Boost your Immune System" by Jennifer Meek & Patrick Holford (1998)
"The Penguin Encyclopaedia of Nutrition" by John Yudkin (1985)
Also you can look up food and energy, fat and insulin on the Internet.

KEY POINTS FROM CHAPTER 2
- Everything we eat is a carbohydrate, fat or protein or a combination of two or all three of these.
- Although we can make energy from carbohydrate, fat or protein, carbohydrates are the easiest foods from which to get fuel.
- When we eat carbohydrates our body decides how much of the energy is needed immediately and how much should be stored for future requirements.
- If our energy storage area (glycogen) is full, insulin will convert the excess to fatty tissue. This is why insulin has been called the fattening hormone.
- If you become diabetic and your body stops producing insulin, or if you stop insulin production with a zero carbohydrate diet, you lose weight dramatically. If a diabetic injects insulin or if you stimulate insulin production with a high carbohydrate diet your weight goes back up. Insulin is an incredibly powerful hormone and has a key role to play in weight control.
- As only carbohydrates trigger the release of insulin, the secret to weight loss lies with carbohydrates.
- The sugar handling mechanism in the body is incredibly sophisticated and complex. It was not designed to cope with the breads, cakes, biscuits and confectionery that we eat today.

PART 2

THE DEFINITION OF MADNESS

PART 2

THE DEFINITION OF MADNESS

Introduction

Someone once told me that the definition of madness is "*doing the same thing again and again and expecting a different result*"!

How many more fad diets or calorie controlled diets do you need to start on Monday and break by Wednesday to convince yourself that this is not the answer? You have to do something different, break the pattern, dare to do something that seems a bit scary to change the results you have had so far. One of the most important things you need to do is to read this section of the book over and over again until you believe it. If you don't challenge some fundamental beliefs that you currently hold to be true you may as well throw away this book and carry on doing what you have been doing and, dare I say, stay overweight for ever. The four myths that you need to throw away are:

- Calorie counting works   WRONG!
- Sugar is OK   WRONG!
- Fat is the enemy   WRONG!
- Fad diets work   WRONG!

28

3

YOU MAY AS WELL COUNT STARS

Why calorie counting doesn't work

How can we say calorie counting doesn't work?

In 1930, two American Doctors, Newburgh and Johnson, published some research that stated "*obesity results from a diet too high in calories.*" Despite the fact that their research was quite limited and they themselves had reservations about the widespread adoption of their original findings, their work remains the basis for slimming advice world-wide.

We should note up front that calorie counting does work but only *in the short term*. Reducing our food intake, below the level that we need, will lead to weight loss *in the short term*. The problem is that in the long term our bodies adjust to the continued starvation and the weight loss slows or even stops altogether. Then, our bodies need less food to survive on a daily basis, so, if we go back to eating the same food we ate before the low calorie diet we will actually put on weight. When we say calorie counting doesn't work, therefore, we are saying that it doesn't work *in the long term*. Calorie counting sends you into a vicious circle of eating less and less just to stay at the same weight.

The calorie theory states that a calorie is "*a unit of heat and energy equal to the amount of heat energy needed to raise the temperature of 1g of water by 1°C from 14.5°C to 15.5°C.*" The theory also states that an average male needs around 3000 calories a day to live and an average female around 2000 calories a day. Finally, the theory tells us if we have a deficit of 3500 calories we will lose 1lb. So the theory tells us to eat fewer calories than our body needs so that we can lose 1lb for every 3500 calories we deprive ourselves of. Here are five reasons why this is simply wrong:

1) People in concentration camps, doing hard physical labour all day long, on a daily intake of around 800 calories would lose approximately a pound a day. A 12st (168lb) male would be 6st (84lb) within twelve weeks and if this didn't kill him he would be 0lb after a further twelve weeks. This is complete nonsense. Clearly no

one would become weightless after twenty four weeks so this theory cannot be true. What will happen is that the 12st male will lose weight rapidly but his miraculous body will then adjust to the food deprivation and adapt to having fewer calories. The weight loss will slow and eventually stop and the body's ability to survive will win through. The calorie theory may have some truth in the short term, but our metabolism soon adjusts and we adapt to having fewer calories to ensure our survival.

2) As we all know from our own experience, we can change our calorie intake significantly and achieve results in the short term but, as time goes on, it becomes increasingly difficult to lose weight. The calorie theory doesn't allow for this – it simply says that if we have a deficit of 3500 calories we will lose a pound. The calorie theory, therefore, makes no distinction between the pounds lost at the start of a diet or the last few pounds to lose, to achieve our goal weight. We know that this is nonsense. We all know that the first seven pounds are so much easier to lose than the last.

3) The calorie theory assumes that it would be physically impossible to lose more than a pound a day. An average man needs around 3000 calories a day, so even if he eats nothing for twenty-four hours he should have a calorie deficit of 3000 and, therefore, lose less than a pound. An average woman needs fewer calories and, therefore, should only lose around half a pound eating nothing for twenty-four hours. Yet we all know when we have been ill, or starved ourselves, we can get on the scales and be anything up to half a stone lighter the next day. It is not uncommon to be 2-3lb lighter. This is all water, they say, but who cares? We are 55-60% water anyway so what else are we going to lose? If we can fit into that party outfit after a day's starvation and a 3lb drop on the scales we don't care what has come off. The calorie theory just doesn't work in practice.

4) You wouldn't be reading this book if calorie counting did work! We have all tried low calorie diets and we now find we can no longer lose weight. 95% of people who have lost weight on a low calorie diet put it back on within months and often more than they originally lost. If it really were as simple as 'eat less than your body needs and you will lose weight', we would have managed it years ago.

5) The calorie theory assumes a direct relationship between calorie deficit and weight loss and this is just not the case. There is a direct relationship in the very short term, but it does not hold over time. The more we cut calories, the greater the deficit we need to lose one more

pound. Our bodies have an incredible survival instinct and, as we try to starve them, our metabolisms adjust to enable us to survive on fewer calories a day. This means that over time we have to eat less and less just to stay the same weight, let alone to lose weight. For many life-long dieters the body just doesn't respond any more to calorie controlled diets.

There was a study in the 1940s by the University of Minnesota. A group of psychologically healthy men of normal weight were put on a diet that, like many currently popular diets, cut their daily calorie intake in half. The men were closely monitored and, over a twelve week period, they lost significant amounts of weight. The average rate at which their bodies digested food also dropped by 40% because their bodies believed that they were experiencing famine. When the diet finished, it took, on average, fourteen months for the men's weight and metabolism to return to normal. During that period, every single one of the men displayed anorexic, bulimic or binge-eating behaviour. They had distorted their bodies' natural weight regulation mechanism and their metabolic systems were out of control. They regained the weight that they had lost, plus about 10% extra and the first weight that they gained was in the form of fat, not muscle.

Most dieters today would panic if they gained back the weight they'd lost and another 10% on top. In fact, most dieters today do panic, because that's exactly what happens to most of them when they stop dieting. And, when people are alarmed, they tend to take drastic action – like starting another diet when the balance of their metabolism is still disturbed from the last one.

I know that this may contradict everything that you have been told over many years but it is so important that you accept that counting calories does not work, in the long run, before moving on. It will take a transformation of your previous thinking habits to be successful from now on in the dieting war. For years you have been taught to count calories and reduce your calorie intake below what you should eat for health and energy. You have gone hungry, you have viewed fat as the devil. You have eaten bland, tasteless foods. You have been deprived. You have probably had some success, only to put weight back on. Or you are a relatively slim person at the moment but you are reading this book to escape the constant battle of bingeing and starving. Or you may be at the point where you just cannot face depriving yourself one more day.

There is an alternative, but you have to completely throw out all your thinking about calories. Keep re-reading this section and convince yourself that the calorie theory is false. If counting calories worked you wouldn't be reading this book! Just hang onto that thought. I have worked with so many people who couldn't let go of counting calories when they started the healthy eating plan in this book. They were terrified of eating fat and they thought they would lose control if quantities were not restricted. Don't hang onto a lie that has not served you well in the past and has made you fatter and less able to lose weight today. Remember that definition of madness – doing the same thing again and again and expecting a different result. You have to try something different, so keep reading and keep that mind open.

I have had many case studies for this eating plan and they also started off as calorie theory devotees. They felt that if they didn't count calories they would overeat and gain weight. In fact they found the exact opposite. They ate more, lost the cravings and gained control over their eating in a way they never imagined possible. You can too...

In Chapter 7 you will read more on not only why calorie counting doesn't work but why it will actually make you fat.

KEY POINTS FROM CHAPTER 3
- Calorie counting doesn't work.
- If the calorie theory did work, we would weigh nothing if we stuck to a low calorie diet for long enough.
- The calorie theory states that a deficit of 3500 calories equals a 1lb weight loss. We all know all people and all pounds are not the same, therefore, this theory cannot be right.
- The theory would mean it would be impossible to lose a pound in a day – we know that this is not true.
- We know calorie counting doesn't work (in the long term) as we have proved this ourselves over and over again. If we do lose weight, we put it back on. Or we can't lose weight without having to cut calories to a seriously low level.
- Our bodies are too clever to be fooled by the calorie theory. When we give them less food than they need (the definition of a calorie controlled diet) they simply adjust to need less food to preserve us and keep us alive.

4

"PURE, WHITE & DEADLY"

Sugar – the more accessible heroin

The title of this chapter is the title of a ground breaking book written by Professor John Yudkin and published in 1972. Professor Yudkin has written many works on sugar and nutrition and his accounts of how he has been attacked by the sugar industry for this are worthy of a John Grisham novel.

World sugar consumption was approximately 130 million tonnes in 2000/01 and is forecast to be 137 million tonnes by 2005. At 8-9 US cents per pound this equates to a sugar industry worth approximately $25 billion world-wide. 65% of the world's sugar is consumed by the developed countries. Understandably the industry didn't like an academic pointing out that their product is *"Pure, White & Deadly."*

However, there are some things about sugar that we should know:

- Sugar can upset blood glucose balance. If we ate sugar cane, like pandas do, we would probably find that our pancreas released an appropriate amount of insulin to cope with the whole food that had been eaten. However, all the sugar we eat in cakes, sweets, chocolate, biscuits, soups, sauces etc. is not the whole cane, but the refined part. It can, therefore, upset our pancreas and our blood glucose level as the body tends to release more insulin than it needs to when we consume sugar and sugar laden foods. This in turn leads to our blood glucose level dropping lower than it was before we ate the sugar, which starts us on a roller coaster of sugar cravings and high and low blood glucose.

- Sugar has practically no nutritional value whatsoever. It is probably the only food or drink that we consume that has no nutritional value. It has no vitamins and barely detectable traces of minerals. There is a table on the next page that compares two apples with approximately a quarter of a litre of milk and 10 teaspoons of sugar – all providing the same number of calories but with very different nutritional values. There are other vitamins and minerals present in milk and apples, which are not shown in the table but everything contained in sugar is shown. As you can see there is no real nutritional benefit from eating sugar.

	Apples (2)	Whole milk (0.2725 litre)	White sugar (10 teaspoons)	Units
Calories	163	163	163	Kj
Potassium	317.0	402.9	0.8	mg
Sodium	0.0	130.3	0.4	mg
Calcium	19.3	317.6	0.4	mg
Folate	7.1	13.2	-	µg
Iron	0.5	0.1	-	mg
Magnesium	13.8	35.8	-	mg
Phosphorus	19.3	248.4	0.8	mg
Vitamin A	13.8	82.5	-	µg
Vitamin B6	0.1	0.1	-	mg
Vitamin C	15.7	2.5	-	mg
Vitamin E	1.6	0.3	-	mg
Zinc	0.1	1.0	-	mg

Source – Encarta Encyclopaedia

- Sugar's calories are empty calories. Because sugar has no nutritional value, when you consume calories from sugar you are not giving your body any of the vitamins and minerals that it needs. Our bodies naturally crave nutrients that we are lacking. Hence any 'empty calories' that we consume are not contributing to our nutritional quotas – they are simply giving us calories and many of us already get more of these than we need.

- Sugar is an anti-nutrient. Worse than not giving you vitamins and minerals, sugar actually depletes your vitamin and minerals. As sugar uses vitamins and minerals in its digestion, and gives none back, it actually makes you worse off than before eating it.

- Sugar is the worst carbohydrate to eat. One carbohydrate is not the same as every other. The sugar manufacturers and confectionery companies like you to think that a carbohydrate is a carbohydrate. They try to tell us that we need calories to survive and for energy and fuel and that carbohydrates play an important part in our diet. Carbohydrates are important as part of our food intake but there is a huge difference between carbohydrates. Take 100g of brown rice and

100g of sugar for example. One provides vitamins and minerals and fibre as well as energy (calories). The other just provides calories. We do need carbohydrates, we do need fuel, we do need energy but there is **always** a better way to consume carbohydrates, fuel and energy than by eating sugar. There is no substance that we eat or drink, which provides fewer nutrients than sugar for the same energy.

- Sugar can make you fat. The sugar manufacturers will tell you that sugar has only 15-20 calories per teaspoon. What they don't tell you is:
    - that your blood glucose level will be affected by the consumption of sugar.
    - that insulin will be released to try to return your blood glucose level to normal and that insulin will affect your weight control.
    - that your pancreas will almost certainly not release the correct amount of insulin to cope with the 'foreign' substance of sugar and, therefore, your blood glucose level may actually end up lower than before you ate the sugar. This can lead to increased cravings for more sugar or anything sweet you can get your hands on.

- Sugar tastes sweet. What's the problem here you may wonder? Well, sugar tastes *so* sweet that it affects our taste buds for naturally sweet foods such as fruit and vegetables. We get to the point where only a confectionery bar will do – apples and carrots just seem bland in comparison. This then leads us to eat more sugar as we get to like the taste.

So many people say, "*Oh I hardly eat sugar*" but they are so wrong. If you think that you don't put sugar in your drinks and, therefore, you don't consume that much, try going through your larder and check each label for sugar (other key words to look for are sucrose, treacle, glucose syrup, dextrose, corn syrup, maltose, anything ending in "*ose*"). Try going round a supermarket one day and seeing exactly which foods contain sugar or other derivatives. The ingredients are listed in order of their presence so you can also see how much sugar is in each food. You will find that most cereals are at least 20% sugar. Almost all sauces, salad dressings and prepared foods contain sugar. Try buying a loaf of bread that doesn't contain sugar, treacle or glucose syrup.

Articles in the national press in the UK in April 2002 reported that the British are eating 1.25lb of sugar per person per week – an increase of 31% in two decades. Over the same period, the number of bags of sugar sold has continually fallen so people are eating more sugar in processed foods they consume rather than using bought sugar in drinks and baking.

The average can of cola contains seven teaspoons of sugar, a leading brand of low fat biscuits was 46% sugar and Slim-Fast is 62% sugar – the articles reported. The Sugar Bureau, the sugar industry's trade association in the UK, counter-claimed *"there is no evidence that high sugar consumption is related to obesity."* Why then are the Americans, who substitute sugar for fat in every processed food imaginable, one of the fattest nations on earth?

I spoke to a Nutritional Advisor at Slim-Fast, in an attempt to understand the high concentration of sugar in a 'diet' food. She explained that as Slim-Fast is a meal replacement product there are strict government guidelines about the content of the product. It must be between 25% and 50% protein, have a maximum of 30% fat and the rest must be carbohydrate. As most slimmers would not want anywhere near 30% fat, even if the maximum protein of 50% is put into a meal replacement, this still leaves up to 50% of the product to be filled up and the only substance left to put in is carbohydrate. (Remember – all foods fall into the categories of carbohydrate, fat and protein). Hence Slim-Fast has no option but to have a high proportion of their product as carbohydrate. They could hardly put potatoes, rice or pasta in a Slim-Fast shake drink so about the only option they have, to make up the 100% with carbohydrate, is sugar. There are three different kinds of sugar in the milk shake meal replacements – sucrose (sugar as we know it), lactose (milk sugar) and maltose.

This is a really key point worth noting in relation to low fat diets – as the only things that we eat are carbohydrate, fat and protein, if you put yourself on a low fat diet and reduce fat as a percentage of your diet, by definition the percentage of one, or both, of the other two needs to go up to compensate. If you eat less fat as a percentage of your diet the percentage of protein and/or carbohydrate in your diet must rise. Add to this the fact that most people on low fat diets also cut back on protein because this often has high fat levels (eggs, meat, oily fish etc) and you can see that people on low fat diets make the primary part of their diet carbohydrates. Think about it – the low calorie (low fat) slimmers' staple foods are fruit, salads, low fat cereal, crisp-breads, rice cakes, sometimes bread or baked potatoes – all high carbohydrate foods. With processed foods, when fat is taken out to make the food 'low fat', one of the most common substances used to replace the fat is sugar. As the Slim-Fast advisor said *"We have to use sugar to fill up the product and to make it palatable!"*

(There are two pie charts in the next chapter to demonstrate what happens to the percentage of carbohydrate in your diet when you try to cut back on fat).

The single best change that you could make to your health and eating, as a result of reading this book, would be to never eat sugar again. It has no nutritional value. You will lose nothing nutritionally by giving it up (in fact you will gain by eating any food in its place as anything else will be more nutritious). Your blood glucose level will be given the chance to stabilise and your cravings will be greatly eased by this. You probably eat sugar currently because it is almost impossible to avoid as it is in so many products. Also you may well crave sugar as it is in the most commonly craved foods – chocolate, ice cream, sweets, biscuits, cakes, muffins – as well as in almost every processed food you can possibly buy.

What else can I read if I want to know more?

"Eat yourself slim" by Michel Montignac (1999)
"Sugar Blues" by William F Duffy (1975)
"Pure White & Deadly" by John Yudkin (1972, 1986)

KEY POINTS FROM CHAPTER 4
- Sugar is the substance to avoid, not fat.
- Sugar can upset blood glucose balance.
- Sugar has practically no nutritional value whatsoever.
- Sugar's calories are empty calories.
- Sugar is an anti-nutrient.
- Sugar is the worst carbohydrate to eat.
- Sugar can make you fat.
- Sugar tastes so sweet it affects our taste buds for natural sweetness.

5

EATING FAT DOESN'T MAKE YOU FAT

Fat is not the enemy – let it be your friend

What is fat?

We described fat in Chapter 2 in the simplest possible way by saying that fat comes from two sources:
1) Animal fat (generally solid at room temperature) – meat, fish, cheese, eggs and dairy foods.
2) Vegetable fat (generally liquid at room temperature) – peanut oil, olive oil, sunflower oil and margarine.

The much more useful categorisation of fat is as follows:
- **Saturated fats** are usually solid, or almost solid, at room temperature. All animal fats, such as those in meat, poultry and dairy products, are saturated. Processed and fast foods are also saturated. Vegetable oils can be saturated. Palm, palm kernel and coconut oils are saturated vegetable oils.

- **Monounsaturated fats** typically remain liquid, even at extremely low temperatures. These fats are found in vegetable oils such as olive oil, peanut oil and canola oil.

- **Polyunsaturated fats** are usually liquid at room temperature. Polyunsaturated fats are found in vegetable oils such as corn oil, safflower oil, soya bean oil and sunflower oil. They are also present in fish and fish oils.

- **Transunsaturated fats** do not occur naturally. In an attempt to make polyunsaturated fats more versatile, the food industry hydrogenates (adds hydrogen atoms to) vegetable oil to make it a more solid fat for the production of margarine and shortenings, as examples. Hence, these fats are also called hydrogenated fats. Manufacturers use this process to increase product stability and shelf life. Thus, a larger quantity can be produced at one time, saving the manufacturer money. Unfortunately, this money-saving process is what contributes to elevated blood cholesterol levels and increased heart disease risk.

Why do we need fat?

Fats serve four key purposes:

1) They provide Essential Fatty Acids (EFA's). There are two EFA's – Omega 6 (linoleic acid) and Omega 3 (linolenic acid). They both derive their names from linseed oil which contains these fatty acids.

2) They are the carriers of the fat soluble vitamins A, D, E and K.

3) They supply the most concentrated form of energy in our diets: 1 gram of fat supplies 9 calories, compared with 7 calories for 1 gram of alcohol and 4 calories for 1 gram of protein or carbohydrate.

4) They help make our diets palatable. Food with little or no fat can be quite tasteless and sometimes difficult to digest.

Fats are crucial for every aspect of our well-being as they form the membrane (protective wall) that surrounds every cell in our bodies. With the right fats our cells are strong, without them they are weak and prone to attack. There are significant deficiency symptoms that arise from not getting enough fat as we will see below.

Are there good fats and bad fats?

There is a lot of literature that categorises fats into good fats and bad fats. There is even a book written called "*Fats that Heal, Fats that Kill*" by Dr Udo Erasmus. When looking at good fats and bad fats the categories of saturated fat, polyunsaturated fat, monounsaturated fat and transunsaturated fat are generally used. It is important to note that many fats are made up of more than one category of fat but they are predominantly one or another. For example olive oil is predominantly a monounsaturated fat, sunflower oil is predominantly a polyunsaturated fat. The following is the composition of a few different types of fats and oils just to give you some examples:

Type of Oil:	Saturated Fat (OK in moderation)	Polyunsaturated Fat (Generally good)	Monounsaturated Fat (Good)
Canola	7%	32%	61%
Coconut	91%	2%	7%
Olive	15%	10%	75%
Peanut	19%	33%	48%
Soya bean	15%	62%	23%
Sunflower	12%	72%	16%

Are we eating enough fat?

a) How can we tell if we are deficient in Essential Fatty Acids?

OMEGA 6 (Linoleic Acid)	OMEGA 3 (Alpha Linolenic Acid)
Omega 6 oils come exclusively from seeds and their oils – hemp, pumpkin, sunflower, sesame, walnut, soya bean and wheat germ.	Omega 3 oils come from linseed, hemp and pumpkin seeds/oils and also oily fish such as mackerel, tuna, salmon and herrings.
Deficiency Symptoms: - Growth retardation - Eczema-like skin conditions - Behavioural disturbances - Arthritis-like conditions - Loss of hair - Liver and kidney degeneration - Excessive water loss through the skin accompanied by thirst - Drying up of glands - Susceptibility to infections - Wounds fail to heal - Sterility in males - Miscarriage in females - Heart and circulatory problems	Deficiency Symptoms: - Growth retardation - Dry skin - Behavioural changes - Tingling sensations in arms and legs - Weakness - Impairment of vision and learning ability - High triglycerides (fats in the blood) - High blood pressure - Sticky platelets - Tissue inflammation - Mental deterioration - Low metabolic rate

b) How can we tell if we are deficient in the fat soluble vitamins?

There are four fat soluble vitamins – A, D, E and K:

1) Deficiency in Vitamin A can lead to night blindness, kidney stones, defective teeth & gums, increased susceptibility to infections and rough, dry, scaly skin.

2) Deficiency in Vitamin D can lead to tooth decay, muscular weakness and a softening of the bones (rickets) which can cause bone fractures or poor healing of fractures.

3) Deficiency in Vitamin E can lead to dry skin, poor muscular & circulatory function, the death of red blood cells and an inability of the white blood cells to resist infection.

4) Deficiency in Vitamin K can lead to diarrhoea and excessive bleeding in the stomach.

Fat – myths and the PR war

The public relations campaign to discredit fat has been very successful. The advice to cut dietary fat first appeared in the 1970s when a Congressional Committee on Nutrition and Human Needs worked to establish the first dietary goals for the United States. The advice relied, almost exclusively, upon work by a nutritionist at the Harvard School of Public Health who believed unconditionally in the benefits of reducing fat intake. The resulting report recommended that Americans drop their fat intake from 40% of their calorie intake (the average at that time) to 30%, with only 10% of that as saturated fat. According to Science Magazine, the report justified its position by stating, *"there are no risks that can be identified and important benefits can be expected"* from reducing fat intake. Hence, even though there was no real evidence that dietary fat intake was linked to health, a national report recommended that Americans change their fat intake.

Americans, generally, have reduced their dietary fat intake as a result of these recommendations, even though possible health benefits were never made clear or quantified. It is most likely that this advice has actually led to health problems. Since Americans have cut down on fat, they've turned to carbohydrate to fill the calorie void. (Remember, cut fat and something else has to go up as a percentage of total calorie intake). Americans as a nation have certainly gained weight – far more people are obese now than were at the time this advice was given.

41

You might think that the Food Standards authorities would have changed their advice over the decades, but no. The USDA standards, issued by the United States Department of Agriculture in 1995, referred to a food pyramid, where they showed the number of portions of each food group that they recommended Americans to be eating each day.

They recommended:

- Hardly any fats & oils. *"Use sparingly"* was the exact advice.
- 2-3 portions of dairy products daily,
- 2-3 portions of protein daily (meat, fish, eggs, pulses),
- 2-4 portions of fruit daily,
- 3-5 portions of vegetables daily,
- 6-11 portions of grains (bread, cereal, rice, pasta) daily.

Taking the upper limits of each of these gives you 26 portions of food of which 20 are carbohydrates and just 6 are fat and protein. Even the three dairy product portions could be carbohydrates too, like milk. Hence almost the entire diet advised by the USDA could be carbohydrate. (www.usda.gov)

Fat has become the real baddie in the diet industry in recent years and it is as important to destroy this myth as it is to stop thinking that calories are the key to weight loss. The argument goes that fat has nine calories per gram while protein and carbohydrate only have four each – therefore, we should cut out as much fat as possible from our diets, to reduce the number of calories we consume. There are numerous diet books, cookery books and processed food products encouraging you to cut out fat at every opportunity. But fat has become the enemy because of the calorie theory. So, because the calorie theory is wrong, we also need to re-examine the role of fat as the 'baddie'.

Fat has also been seen as the baddie in weight gain, high cholesterol and heart disease. Let us look at each of these in turn:

Myth 1 – Eating fat makes you fat

Eating fat does not make you fat. **It is your body's response to excess carbohydrates in your diet that makes you fat**. Your body has a limited capacity to store excess carbohydrates, but it can easily convert those excess carbohydrates into excess body fat.

Here are three key reasons why eating fat does *not* make you fat:

1) We have already established that insulin is the fattening hormone and pure fat has no impact on insulin whatsoever. You can eat any high fat, zero carbohydrate food and your body will not pump out any

insulin at all. You can eat steak, pork fat, butter, cream, oily fish, eggs, pure lard if your stomach can take it, and you will not stimulate the production of insulin. This is why high fat/low carbohydrate diets work so well – no matter how many calories you consume you do not stimulate the production of insulin and, therefore, you do not put on weight. In fact quite the opposite happens. If you eat nothing but fat/protein you will actually lose weight rapidly as your body goes into a state known as Ketosis and you burn the fat stored in your body for energy. (Ketosis occurs in situations where the energy being produced by the body has to come from fat rather than from carbohydrate). If you really don't believe this, eat nothing but fat/protein for as long as you can manage – few people can manage more than a few days unless they are stranded in the arctic and have no choice – and see how much weight you lose. Even in just a weekend you could experience dramatic weight loss.

2) The argument for 'eating fat makes you fat' is based on the calorie theory. The idea is that, because fat has more calories per gram than protein or carbohydrate, eating fat will provide more calories and therefore makes us fat. We now know that calorie counting doesn't work so it doesn't matter how many calories fat has compared with protein or carbohydrate because we don't count calories any more. What is important is **what** we eat, not **how much** or **how many calories**.

3) In a study done in 1956 by Professor Kekwick and Dr Pawan, groups of dieters were given the same number of calories, 1000 per day, but the groups were given very different compositions of carbohydrate, fat and protein. One diet was 90% carbohydrate, another 90% fat, another 90% protein and the final one was a more typical balanced diet with all three. Those on the high fat diet lost the most, those on the high carbohydrate diet lost the least. Some even put weight on with the high carbohydrate diet! In further tests, calories from fat and protein were increased to almost 3000 per day – but with carbohydrate still severely restricted – and the group continued to lose weight. This supported other findings in the USA around the same time where it was demonstrated that the greater the amount of fat in the diet the greater the weight loss.

It is essential to remember, however, that the above applies to eating fat on its own. If you eat fat at the same time as carbohydrate, the body will use the carbohydrate for energy and store the fat as fatty tissue.

Myth 2 – Eating fat increases cholesterol

Cholesterol is found in all animal products – meat, fish, seafood, eggs and dairy products. It is especially high in egg yolks and organ meats, such as liver, brains and kidneys. Eating foods high in cholesterol tends to raise the level of cholesterol in our bodies. The National Cholesterol Education Program recommends eating fewer than 300mg of cholesterol per day.

Vegetable products do not contain cholesterol, but they may be loaded with fat, which in turn affects our cholesterol levels. Labels stating "*No Cholesterol*" on food packages should alert you to look at the nutritional information to determine the exact amount of fat and saturated fat. Research has shown that saturated fat is the strongest determinant of blood cholesterol levels (more than actually eating cholesterol itself).

So, some fat increases cholesterol, other fat doesn't. We now know that there is 'good' cholesterol and there is 'bad' cholesterol. The key thing is to increase, or at least keep neutral, the good cholesterol and to reduce, or at least keep neutral, the bad cholesterol. The table below summarises the effect of the four different types of fat on cholesterol. If you take saturated fat, for example, this has no effect on good cholesterol which is OK. It raises bad cholesterol which is not OK. So, its overall effect on cholesterol is negative. It is not as bad as transunsaturated fat, however, which lowers the good cholesterol, increases the bad cholesterol and is, therefore, the worst fat of all.

FAT	GOOD CHOLESTEROL (HDL)	BAD CHOLESTEROL (LDL)	OVERALL IMPACT ON CHOLESTEROL
Transunsaturated	Lowers it – Not OK	Raises it – Not OK	Very bad
Saturated	No effect – OK	Raises it – Not OK	Bad
Polyunsaturated	Lowers it – Not OK	Lowers it – OK	Mixed on cholesterol but provides EFA's
Monounsaturated	No effect – OK	Lowers it – OK	Good

The fats we should totally avoid, therefore, are transunsaturated fats:
- They lower HDL (good) cholesterol, raise LDL (bad) cholesterol and raise overall cholesterol. They also increase Lp(a) levels which are a particularly bad form of cholesterol and they raise triglyceride levels which are fats found in the blood.

- Transunsaturated fats are found in margarine, manufactured fats, shortening and anywhere where you see the description 'hydrogenated' fats.

The fats we should eat with caution, therefore, are Saturated fats:
- These raise LDL (bad) and total cholesterol, though they have no impact on good cholesterol.
- Saturated fats are found in animal foods like meat and dairy products.

The fats we need, therefore, are:
- Polyunsaturated fats which lower bad cholesterol and provide the Essential Fatty Acids Omega 3 and Omega 6. These are found in seeds and their oils and fish and their oils.
- Monounsaturated fats which lower overall cholesterol. These are found in olive oil and canola oil.

Myth 3 – Eating fat increases the risk of heart disease

Before 1920 coronary heart disease was rare in America; so rare that when a young doctor imported an electrocardiograph, his colleagues at Harvard University advised him to concentrate on a more profitable branch of medicine. By the mid fifties heart disease was the leading cause of death among Americans and today it causes at least 40% of all deaths in the US.

If, as has been claimed, heart disease results from the consumption of saturated fat, we would expect to find a corresponding increase in animal fat in the American diet. In fact the reverse is true. During the sixty-year period from 1910 to 1970, the proportion of traditional animal fat in the American diet declined from 83% to 62%, and butter consumption fell from 18lb per person per year to 4. Since the 1920s dietary cholesterol intake has increased by only 1%. What has increased over the past eighty years, however, is the proportion of vegetable oils in the form of margarine, shortening and refined oils in our diet. These have increased approximately 400% and the consumption of sugar and processed foods has increased by about 60%.

The National Centre for Biotechnology Information published a study in November 2002 by S. Renaud and D. Lanzmann-Petithory called *"Dietary Fats and Coronary Heart Disease."* This study found that when the consumption of saturated fat was reduced and replaced, in part, with unsaturated omega-6 fats, there was no decrease in heart disease. It was only when Omega 3 fatty acids were added to the diet that fatal and nonfatal heart attacks were significantly lowered. This implies that eating good fat is of more benefit than cutting saturated fat in the effort to cut heart disease.

The National Institute of Health has now recommended that fat intake should not be reduced below 30% of total calories consumed. They further advise that having monounsaturated and polyunsaturated fats, instead of saturated and hydrogenated fats, will improve both health and longevity. They interestingly conclude that extremely low fat diets are probably dangerous.

The PR on fat has started to change, but it may take years to reverse the bad image that people have in their minds. Science magazine has recently reported that there are no studies to show a clear and compelling link between high levels of dietary fat and heart disease or risk of heart attack. There will need to be far more positive messages about fat, however, before beliefs will really change.

A really important point...

The key thing to note is that fat is not the enemy for the simple reason that if you reduce fat in your diet you have to replace it with something else. If you imagine your food intake as a pie diagram adding up to one hundred, if your food intake has previously been carbohydrate 45%, fat 35% and protein 20% then, if your fat intake goes down, the carbohydrate percentage has to go up. (Most protein is also fat so people following low fat diets invariably cut back on both fat and protein).

This pie chart below shows a moderate fat diet with carbohydrate at 45%, fat at 35% and protein at 20%

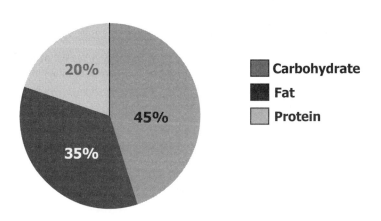

Moderate Fat Diet

The next diagram shows what happens when someone switches from a 'normal' diet to a low fat diet (i.e. when they start counting calories).

Low Fat Diet

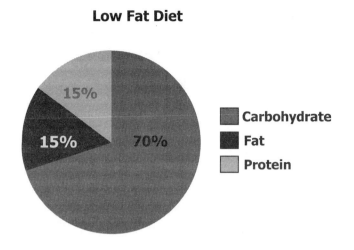

In the second pie chart above, the percentage of fat goes down from 35% to 15%. The percentage of protein goes down from 20% to 15% but the percentage of carbohydrate goes *up* from 45% to 70%. These are just example numbers but they do clearly show that, when people try to cut fat in their diet, the only thing that can go up to compensate for this is the percentage of carbohydrate. Low fat diets, therefore, are, by definition, high carbohydrate diets. You may not think of fruits, vegetables, salads and low fat meals as high in carbohydrate but they are.

Knowing what we now know about insulin, the increased carbohydrate consumption will stimulate the production of insulin, the fattening hormone. The fat and protein that you were eating before had no impact on insulin. If you want to lose weight, therefore, you do not want to go on a low fat diet as this is the same as a high carbohydrate diet, which stimulates insulin production, which is what we want to avoid.

When you really understand the way the body deals with food and truly believe that it is insulin, not calories, which makes you fat, then you will know not to avoid calories or fat but to manage the production of insulin instead.

What else can I read if I want to know more?

"The Cholesterol Myths: Exposing the Fallacy that Saturated Fat and Cholesterol cause Heart Disease" by Uffe Ravenskov MD, PhD (2002)
"Know your fats: The Complete Primer for Understanding the Nutrition of Fats, Oils and Cholesterol" by Mary Enig, PhD (2000)
"Fats that Heal, Fats that Kill" by Dr Udo Erasmus (1993)

KEY POINTS FROM CHAPTER 5

- Fat comes from either animal or vegetable sources. Fat is categorised into four groups – saturated fat, monounsaturated fat, polyunsaturated fat and transunsaturated fat.
- We need fat for our health – for skin, nails, eyes and every cell in our bodies. We need fat soluble vitamins and Essential Fatty Acids in our diets and these are found in some of the fats that we eat.
- Simplistically, monounsaturated and polyunsaturated fats are good for you, saturated fats less so and transunsaturated fats not at all.
- Fat has been the subject of a lot of negative PR from within the food industry to the extent that many people actively try to avoid fat in their diet.
- Eating fat does not make you fat. Eating fat at the same time as carbohydrate can make you fat (because the body will use the carbohydrate for energy and store the fat) but fat in itself is not the enemy.
- Not all fat raises cholesterol. Transunsaturated fat raises cholesterol and saturated fat raises cholesterol but monounsaturated fat lowers bad cholesterol and polyunsaturated fat lowers both bad and good cholesterol.
- Monounsaturated and polyunsaturated fats are needed by the body and we cannot get Essential Fatty Acids and fat soluble vitamins without them.
- Cutting fat out of your diet means that the percentage of carbohydrate goes up instead. As fat does not stimulate the production of insulin (the fattening hormone) and carbohydrate does, this is not a good idea.

6

CABBAGE SOUP FOR THE SOUL

You need never try another fad diet again

Balanced diets are better than fad diets

We shouldn't have to devote a chapter to this statement as we know it makes sense. We know that any diet that tells us to eat 90% protein or 90% carbohydrate or 100% liquid cannot be healthy.

We need to get a wide variety of foods to get all the vitamins and minerals that we need for optimal health. We need to eat a balanced diet containing carbohydrate, fat and protein.

We know all of this so why do we follow fad diets? Why do December magazines with "*lose 10lb before Christmas*" sell so well? Why has the Cabbage Soup diet been such a hit? Who has tried the egg and grapefruit diet? Liquid only diets? Meal replacement bars?

We try them because all we want is to be slim.

We will do anything to be slim. We will take diet pills, we will staple our stomachs and have liposuction in the extreme. It should be staggering that we would even consider life-endangering, invasive surgery to be slim, but probably few people reading this are shocked – we can all understand the desperation to be slim.

We have also probably had limited success with fad (crash) diets in the short term. The principle behind any fad diet is almost always dramatic calorie reduction, which will work, in the short term, if followed rigorously. If you can eat nothing but eggs and grapefruit from Monday to Friday you probably will lose a few pounds before that wedding at the weekend. However, at what expense? You will be exhausted, cranky, irritable and as for your skin and breath let's not even think about them!

The liquid diets and meal replacements are all calorie controlled and they ensure your calorie deprivation. Even the hugely popular Scarsdale Medical diet is just a seriously calorie controlled diet. In the opening chapters we are told that the diet averages 1000 calories or fewer per day.

Let us summarise what we know about fad diets:

- They are not balanced,
- They are not a way of life to be followed for any length of time,
- They do not re-educate your eating habits,
- They take the willpower of a monk to stick to,
- You binge as soon as you stop, or give up when you have reached your limit of hunger and deprivation,
- They slow your metabolism and waste lean muscle which then makes it even harder for you to lose weight in the future,
- You are almost certainly overweight today as a result of fad diets followed in the past,
- And perhaps the most important thing of all...

...they don't work!

They may do in the short term, but you know how quickly you put the weight back on and more. They do not work in the long term.

The good news about the eating advice in this book is that you will lose weight as soon as you start the programme. You will also lose weight initially very quickly, especially if you have been suffering from any of the conditions that we will come onto in Part 3. Hence, don't worry about giving up fad diets for a long slow haul instead. You will achieve great results, and you will be delighted at how quickly you will lose weight, but this will not be because you are on a fad diet. It will be because you are listening to your body and giving it what it needs.

If you want a quick fix weight loss at any time, just do the 5 day kick-start eating plan in Chapter 13 and you will lose weight quickly and without feeling hungry. You will also have far more energy and much better breath than on a fad diet.

KEY POINTS FROM CHAPTER 6
- Fad diets do not work in the long term.
- They may work in the short term but they work on the basis of dramatically reducing calorie intake and, therefore, they can make you even fatter in the long term.

PART 3

WHY DO YOU OVEREAT?
WHEN ALL YOU WANT IS TO BE SLIM

PART 3

WHY DO YOU OVEREAT?
WHEN ALL YOU WANT IS TO BE SLIM

Introduction

Why do you overeat? – When all you want is to be slim.

The answer to this question is that you overeat because you have insatiable cravings, which are as difficult to fight as any drug addict's or alcoholic's. The added challenge for you is that you can't go 'cold turkey' on food, in the way a drug user or alcoholic can, to kick their addiction. What we need to answer, therefore, is why you have these insatiable cravings that make your desire for food greater than your desire to be slim at the key moment when you overeat.

There is one thing that you are doing, and there are three conditions that you may be suffering from, which are driving these insatiable cravings.

The one thing that you are doing is calorie counting.

The three conditions are:

1) Candida
2) Food Intolerance
3) Hypoglycaemia

The first part of this section explains why calorie counting has made you fat and why it will continue to do so for as long as you do it. We then go on to look at each of the three conditions above – Candida, Food Intolerance and Hypoglycaemia – to show how they lead to insatiable cravings.

A point worth making at this stage of the book is that you may not be suffering from the three conditions discussed in Part 3. You may have recently decided that you want to lose weight, and have heard how easy and effective this eating plan is, and you may have a relatively strong immune system at this stage. You may have been calorie counting for only a short period of time and have not exposed yourself too much to the causes of Candida, Food Intolerance and Hypoglycaemia.

If you read through Part 3 and do not empathise with many, or any, of the symptoms described then you should be delighted. You have found the right eating plan before it is too late and you will be able to follow the rules in Chapter 14 with relative ease compared to the advanced food addicts. Please do read Part 3, however, as you may well find that you are suffering from one of the conditions that we are about to explore. If you crave sugar and bread you may well have Candida. If you have one particular food or food group that you crave, you may well have Food Intolerance. If you have blood glucose highs and lows throughout the day, you may well have Hypoglycaemia.

Dr David Williams, author of *"Hypoglycaemia: The Deadly Roller Coaster"*, estimates that as many as 100 million Americans could be suffering from Hypoglycaemia. This represents approximately 40% of the US population and is likely to be replicated at this level elsewhere in the developed world.

It is also estimated that approximately 100 million people in the US may be affected by *'sick all over syndrome'* with which Candida and Food Intolerance are invariably implicated. Hence, the odds would strongly suggest that you do have one or more of the three conditions. So, read on…

7

CALORIE COUNTING MAKES YOU FAT

It doesn't make you slim, it actually makes you fat

It is a frequently documented fact that 95% of people who lose weight on a calorie controlled diet regain that weight. Some research has estimated this figure to be as high as 98%.

You know yourself that calorie counting doesn't work in the long run, otherwise you wouldn't be reading this book.

We saw in Chapter 3 that calorie counting doesn't work. We now show how calorie counting actually makes you fat and here is why…

1) A calorie controlled diet is by definition a diet which ensures that we take in fewer calories than our bodies need on a daily basis. Imagine if you were asked to drive from John O'Groats to Lands End in the UK, or from the West to the East Coast of America, but without putting enough fuel in the car to do so. You would think this was mad and yet millions of people in the 'developed' world are deliberately trying to run their bodies on less fuel than they need, every day. This is the very idea of the calorie controlled diet – take in less fuel than you need. The theory is that your body will make up for the calorie deficit by burning fat that you have stored already, but it is not as simple as this. Your body first and foremost is a survival machine. The human body has developed over thousands of years and it has survived and adapted to far more challenging things than calorie counting. All our natural instincts – the fright, flight, fight mechanism for example – are designed to help us survive. Your whole body is designed to help you survive. When we deny our bodies the fuel that they need, the following happens:

a) Our metabolism slows down so that our bodies adjust to having less fuel. The longer we diet, the more our bodies adjust and the more they adapt to a lower fuel intake.

b) Our bodies store fat – they will fight to hang onto the thing best placed to keep us alive (your body thinks you have been stranded on a desert island – it doesn't realise you have just read a diet book!)

c)   Our bodies will use muscle if they can't get enough fuel and once we have used up this muscle it is very difficult to replace. This is why persistent dieters find themselves getting fatter and fatter every time they regain weight. They have actually regained fat to replace lean muscle lost and fat takes up more room for the same weight than lean muscle. The added insult to injury here is that muscle also boosts the metabolic rate so the more muscle you lose the more your metabolism is adversely affected.

Just to illustrate this, I recall a fitness assessment which was offered at a company where I used to work. An anorexic worked in the same department as me – she was a few inches taller and approximately 30lb lighter but her body fat percentage was several points higher than mine.

So, the conclusion of this first point is that our bodies are way more sophisticated than the calorie theory gives them credit for. If we try to restrict calories, i.e. if we try to take in less fuel than we need, our bodies will adapt in a number of different ways. All of these ways work against us in the long run, either by slowing down our metabolisms or by actively making our bodies store fat.

2) The second point is starving leads to bingeing – for every action there is an equal and opposite reaction. Have you noticed how starving and bingeing go together? The more you starve the more extreme the binges get. It becomes hard to know what causes what. You binge, so you try to starve the next day and you binge because you are so hungry from having starved the day before. It is a vicious circle, which seems so difficult to break out of. The key is to do neither – don't starve and don't binge. Easier said than done? Not if you can break the cravings that make you binge and stop the starving that makes you hungry. Please keep reading…

The opening to this part of the book said that there is one thing that you are doing, and three things from which you may be suffering, which are causing your food cravings. These cravings lead you to overeat when all you want is to be slim. The one thing that you are doing is calorie counting. You have to stop counting calories if you want to be slim in the long term. Don't panic! You won't put on weight if you stop counting calories. You actually need to stop counting calories to lose weight in the long term. It is **what** you eat more than **how much** you eat that is making you fat.

If you remain convinced that calorie counting is the way to long term weight loss then why are you reading this book? You know that calorie counting doesn't work. You've tried it yourself, maybe you have lost weight and then regained it, maybe you have seen friends or colleagues do the same. Remember the definition of madness – doing the same thing again and again and expecting a different result – and ask yourself what you've got to lose by trying something different.

KEY POINTS FROM CHAPTER 7

- Calorie counting not only doesn't work – it makes you fat.
- Our bodies are too clever to be fooled by the calorie theory. When we take in fewer calories than we need, the following happens a) our metabolisms slow down b) our bodies store fat and c) our bodies consume muscle if they can't get enough fuel. Muscle lost is very difficult to replace and it can lead to us getting fatter in the longer term.
- Reactions are equal and opposite – starving leads to bingeing and bingeing leads to starving. The higher the highs we have in life, the lower the lows. Things do go together equally and oppositely. If you try to count calories your body will drive you to overeat. The more you starve the more you binge.

8

"I'M SAM AND I'M A FOOD ADDICT"

Food addiction and food cravings

As we saw in the introduction, addiction to a substance has four main characteristics:

1) An uncontrollable craving.
2) Increasing tolerance so that more of the addictive substance is needed in order to produce the same effects.
3) Physical or psychological dependence – consumption of the substance leads to a feeling of well-being (euphoria in the extreme) at the outset and then, in the latter stages of the addiction, the substance is needed to avoid unpleasant withdrawal symptoms.
4) Adverse effects on the consumer.

We used the example of chocolate to show how these four characteristics applied:

1) First, the uncontrollable cravings…

2) Secondly, the binges get worse and worse and you feel the need to consume ever-increasing quantities of chocolate to satisfy your addiction.

3) Then physical and/or psychological dependence occurs. You feel addicted both physically and mentally – if you go without your fix you get physical symptoms like headaches and psychological symptoms like irritability and an inability to concentrate. Both are an indication of the physical and psychological dependence. You reach the point where you no longer get good feelings when you consume chocolate but you actually need chocolate to stop the withdrawal symptoms. i.e. you need the substance not to feel good but to stop feeling bad.

4) Finally, think about the adverse effects that you get when you eat chocolate (or whatever the food is that you most crave) – the

unbearable cravings, the dopey feelings, headaches, bloating, weight gain/fluctuations, fatigue... the list is endless.

We also said in the introduction that food addiction differs from drug addiction only in the extreme lengths people will go to for their fix and perhaps in the strength of the adverse effects. In general drug addiction leads to more physical and mental damage than food addiction but if you have seen a 200-300lb person with no energy or health or desire for life, existing day to day rather than living, you may wonder that there is little difference in the effect that food or heroin can have on our well-being. Drug addicts will commit crime for their fix but maybe this is only because of the price of the substance. If chocolate cost hundreds of dollars for an ounce what would addicts do to get their fix? I have heard chocolate addicts joke that they would *'mug an old lady'* for a confectionery bar – perhaps there is a dark undercurrent to the joke!

So how do we overcome this? What does food addiction tell us about why we are overeating? The message for overcoming overeating is this – you will continue to overeat, that is to crave food uncontrollably, unless you identify and avoid all foods to which you are addicted. I'll repeat this again as it really is so important – **you will continue to overeat, that is to crave food uncontrollably, unless you identify and avoid all foods to which you are addicted**.

You overeat and binge compulsively because you have one, or all, of a number of conditions which we focus on at length in this part of the book. There are three conditions which lead to immense food cravings and they are Candida, Food Intolerance and Hypoglycaemia. You may have one, or all, of these conditions and any, or all, of them will lead to addict-like cravings. You are not weak willed. You are not greedy. You have a health problem, or a number of health problems, and you must think of yourself like a diabetic in that there are certain foods that you simply must avoid for your health. You are an alcoholic with food in place of alcohol. You are a nicotine addict with food in place of cigarettes.

Unfortunately, however, in many ways, your problem is worse. An alcoholic can overcome their problem by avoiding alcohol altogether. A nicotine addict must give up cigarettes. A drug addict must stop taking drugs. You, a food addict, cannot stop eating. You have to learn to live with food and to eat in such a way that you don't binge and, most importantly, that you don't have an uncontrollable desire to binge. There is a way to do this...

You don't stop eating, but you do stop eating the foods that contribute to the conditions that are causing your cravings. We will see in the rest of this section how to identify the conditions you may be suffering from and the foods you, therefore, need to avoid. The good news is that many of the conditions are caused by having a weakened immune system and they further weaken the immune system, in a vicious circle, once they take hold. Hence, if you can break out of the vicious circle and start improving your immune system you will be able to re-introduce foods in the future which are currently causing you problems. You must stop eating the foods that are making you overeat and overweight **now,** but you won't have to give them up for ever.

In the following sections on Candida, Food Intolerance and Hypoglycaemia there are explicit passages from many books which refer to addict-like food cravings. These books all identify specific food cravings as cardinal signs of Candida, Food Intolerance and Hypoglycaemia. Yet such information remains exclusive to books on these conditions and is rarely found in books on eating disorders. Why? We are led to believe that eating disorders are psychological disorders and not physical disorders. However, the medical evidence for food cravings, in relation to Candida, Food Intolerance and Hypoglycaemia, seems indisputable and the overeater can benefit so much from being aware of the physical factors that may be causing their irrational behaviour.

KEY POINTS FROM CHAPTER 8

- Addiction has four distinct characteristics – 1) an uncontrollable craving, 2) a need to consume ever-increasing quantities of the substance to satisfy the addiction, 3) the occurrence of physical and/or psychological dependence and 4) the substance produces adverse side effects.
- Food addiction is just like cigarette, drug or alcohol addiction. It differs, and then only marginally, in the lengths some people will go to to feed their addiction.
- Alcoholics and drug addicts are advised to go 'cold turkey'. You cannot stop eating food but you can stop eating the foods to which you are addicted.
- You will continue to overeat, to crave food uncontrollably, unless you identify and avoid all foods to which you are addicted.
- Food addiction is very much a physical issue. Overeating can have psychological causes and effects but we should not ignore the physical causes behind it.
- Candida, Food Intolerance and Hypoglycaemia are the three key conditions that cause food addiction.

9

HOW YOUR GUT FLORA ARE MAKING YOU FAT

Candida – everything you need to know

What is Candida?

Candida Albicans is a yeast that exists in all of us which is normally controlled by our immune system and by other bacterial flora present in our body. It usually resides in the digestive tract and is observed in females in the vagina, or in any sufferer on the skin (athlete's foot or dandruff, for example, are generally signs of fungal or yeast infections). Candida serves no useful purpose in the body (unlike other bacterial flora such as lactobacillus acidophilus) and can, therefore, be viewed as a parasite. In many people this yeast causes no harm and lives within them peacefully. The problem starts when Candida gets out of control and does make its presence known.

Yeast exists just about everywhere on earth, living off other living things. In the right environment, yeast is capable of explosive reproduction and growth, as anyone who has ever made bread, wine or beer will know. Science has shown that a single yeast cell, given the right reproductive environment, can multiply to over one hundred yeast cells within twenty-four hours. In the human body, therefore, given the right environment, this normally harmless yeast can multiply to frightening levels and cause significant impact on our health and well-being.

What causes Candida overgrowth?

Or put another way – if yeast can multiply to frightening levels given the right environment – what makes our body the right environment for Candida to multiply?

There are five key causes:
1) A weakened immune system,
2) Over-consumption of refined carbohydrates,
3) Medication – steroids, antibiotics, birth control pills, hormones,
4) Diabetes,
5) Nutritional deficiency.

1) If you have a weakened immune system you are more susceptible to Candida overgrowth and in fact Candida overgrowth is often seen as evidence of a weakened immune system. One will make the other worse in a vicious circle. If you have had a period of illness, or significant personal or work stress, the chances are that your immune system will be weaker than normal and this provides an ideal opportunity for Candida to multiply. This will then further weaken your immune system.

2) Anyone who has made beer at home will know the effect of combining yeast, sugar and vinegar. The effect on Candida is much the same. The yeast thrives on all refined carbohydrates, concentrated fruit sugar, yeast and yeast derivatives and vinegary/pickled foods. The fact that Candida emerged as a significant health issue in the twentieth century is not surprising given the recent increase in processed food consumption. As we have increased our consumption of refined foods, we have fed the parasite Candida in our body and enabled it to get out of balance. The added harm that we have done, by over consuming refined carbohydrates, is that we have depleted our bodies of nutrients in their digestion without adding many back in return. Sugar is the worst culprit for nutrient depletion as was seen in Chapter 4.

3) There are many modern medicines that upset our natural body harmony and encourage the overgrowth of Candida. These include steroids, antibiotics, birth control pills and hormones, all of which were unknown before the twentieth century. This is a further reason why Candida, and the related obesity problems, have become far more prevalent in recent years. Antibiotics are chemical substances capable of destroying or inhibiting the growth of living things such as germs but they are also capable of killing lactobacilli, which are found in the intestines. Lactobacilli are part of the 'friendly' gut bacteria which control Candida and thus antibiotics can contribute to a proliferation of Candida as the gut flora balance is disturbed.

4) As we know from Chapter 2, diabetes is also known as "*sweet urine*" and it occurs where the pancreas does not release insulin to regulate the glucose level in the blood. Diabetics, who literally have an excess of glucose in their blood, are providing the ideal breeding ground for Candida. It is well know that diabetics struggle more with their weight than the average non-diabetic and there could be a few reasons for this:

- The injections of insulin lead directly to weight problems as insulin is the fattening hormone (remember what we don't use up is stored as fatty tissue).
- Diabetics are more prone to Candida with their sugary body environment and, therefore, the cravings linked to Candida are likely to be making them fat.
- Diabetics don't have a natural mechanism to regulate their blood glucose level and are, therefore, trying to avoid a state of Hypoglycaemia at all times by balancing injections with food consumed. They are, therefore, susceptible to food cravings if this balance is out of sync at any time.

5) There is much evidence to suggest that our nutritional deficiency has actually got worse and not better as we have 'developed' as nations. Analysis in the UK reveals that the war time diet, when food was rationed, was actually better for us than our current diet where we can freely choose from every food available. In war time we were limited to fixed amounts of meat, fish, vegetables, fruits, dairy products and grains but we were also limited in our access to sugar and other refined carbohydrates. In comparison with current diets, high in refined carbohydrates and processed foods, our predecessors ate quite well. We may be overeating as developed nations but we are certainly not over consuming vitamins. A number of nutrients are key to the control of Candida and there is evidence that they are lacking in our current diets:
- Biotin, one of the B vitamins, can help prevent the conversion of the yeast form of Candida to its fungal form. One of the richest sources of biotin is pigs' kidneys while reasonable sources are eggs and whole grains.
- Vitamin C affects general immunity which impacts the environment in which yeast can multiply. Stress also depletes vitamin C and we may not be getting the levels of Vitamin C we need for optimal health and immunity with our current 'fast food' diets. Vitamin C is not stored by the body so we need a constant supply to keep Candida at bay.
- B vitamins are also needed for stress tolerance and the immune system and we lose valuable sources of B vitamins when we opt for refined carbohydrates over whole-meal carbohydrates. Cereals and breads are often fortified with added vitamins and these are the only sources of B vitamins in many of our diets. However, these come in products laden with sugar and other refined carbohydrates so we would be better off avoiding them altogether and eating the whole foods or taking a vitamin pill on its own.

- Magnesium, selenium and zinc are the key minerals needed for the immune system and we generally find that modern diets are deficient in all three of these. Magnesium is found in Soya beans, nuts and whole grains. Selenium is found in kidneys & liver, fish & shellfish and whole grains. Zinc is found in oysters, meat, fish & shellfish and hard cheese. If your diet is lacking in nuts, whole grains, high quality fish, shellfish and meat you may well be lacking in any, or all, of these minerals.

All of the nutritional deficiencies highlighted above can create the environment in which Candida can multiply within us.

How do you know if you have Candida overgrowth?

In general, chronic Candida overgrowth can make a person feel very unwell all over. Here are some of the many symptoms that you may be experiencing if you have Candida overgrowth:

Stomach – constipation; diarrhoea; irritable bowel syndrome; stomach distension; bloating, especially after eating; two sets of clothes needed for pre and post eating; indigestion; gas; heartburn.

Head – headaches; dizziness; earaches; blurred vision; flushed cheeks; feeling of 'sleepwalking'; feeling unreal; feeling 'spaced out'.

Women – Pre-Menstrual Tension (PMT); water retention; irregular menstruation; painful breasts; vaginal discharge or itchiness; thrush; cystitis.

Blood Glucose – hungry between meals; irritable or moody before meals; shaky when hungry; faintness when food is not eaten; irregular pulse before and after eating; headaches late morning; waking in the early hours and not being able to get back to sleep; abnormal cravings for sweet foods, bread, alcohol or caffeine; eating sweets increases hunger; excessive appetite; instant sugar 'high' followed by fatigue; chilly feeling after eating.

Mental – anxiety; depression; irritability; lethargy; memory problems; loss of concentration; moodiness; nightmares; mental 'sluggishness'; "*get up and go*" has got up and gone.

Other – athletes foot; dandruff or other fungal infections; Food Intolerance; dramatic fluctuations in weight from one day to the next; poor circulation; hands and feet sensitive to cold; exhaustion; feeling of being unable to cope; constant fatigue; muscle aches; susceptibility to infection; gasping for breath; sighing often – 'hunger for air'; tightness in chest; chest aches; cramps; yawning easily; insomnia; excessive thirst; easy weight gain; coated tongue; dry skin; hair loss; symptoms worse after consuming yeast or sugary foods; symptoms worse on damp, humid or rainy days.

As you can see, the complaints attributable to Candida are many and varied. If you are feeling very unwell at the moment you may identify with many of the above symptoms and you may be as worried about your general health as you are about your eating habits. However, many readers will be most aware of the sugar handling problems, water retention, fatigue, easy weight gain, dramatic fluctuations in weight, stomach bloating, depression, anxiety and other symptoms common to eating problems. If Candida is left unchecked you could soon develop many of the other symptoms until your health deteriorates to an unprecedented level. Candida does not get better on its own – it gets worse. At the moment you may just be worried about sugar cravings and weight fluctuations but things could get a lot worse.

If you need a further check list to add to the above, the following questionnaire should help you identify if Candida is a problem for you. The questionnaire on the next page shows the **causes** of Candida. If you have many of the things that can cause Candida you may well find that this is a problem for you.

CAUSES	SCORING	POINTS
IMMUNE SYSTEM: (No Maximum) - Have you suffered illness in the past two years, which would indicate a weakened immune system?	1 point for each day 'sick'	5
CARBOHYDRATES: (Maximum 10) - Do you eat refined carbohydrates? (Sugar, white flour, white rice, white pasta, cakes, biscuits, confectionery etc)	1 for each meal/ snack per day, which includes them.	7
- Do you eat more portions of carbohydrates (including fruit) than protein each day?	5 points if yes	5
MEDICATION: (No Maximum) - How many times have you taken antibiotics during childhood?	1 for each occasion	10
- How many times have you taken antibiotics during adulthood?	1 for each occasion	15
- Have you taken birth control pills?	2 for each occasion	4
- Have you taken hormones in any other form?	1 for each occasion	
- Have you taken steroids (e.g. predisone or cortisone)?	1 for each occasion	
- Have you ever been pregnant?	2 for each occasion	
DIABETES: (Maximum 10) - Are you diabetic?	10 if yes	
NUTRITIONAL DEFICIENCY: (Maximum 10) Do you have any signs of nutritional deficiency?	2 for each example	
- White spots on finger nails,		2
- Dry flaky skin or brittle hair or nails,		
- Poor hair or skin condition,		
- Muscle aches or general tiredness,		2
- Dull, dry eyes		2

You could score anywhere between 0 and 200, or even more in really extreme cases (where you have had many days of sickness for example).

The more points you score overall and the more sections out of the five that you score points in; the more likely you are to have Candida as you will be showing strong evidence for the causes of Candida. If you score points in each of the five sections you have been exposed to all the key causes of Candida and, therefore, you will almost certainly be suffering from this condition. You can still be a sufferer scoring in just one or two of the sections.

Having looked at the **causes**, we move onto the **symptoms**. The following questionnaire looks at the symptoms of Candida and whether or not you have an overgrowth of this parasite.

In the following table please score as follows:
- 1 point for each symptom that is occasional and mild,
- 2 points for each symptom that is frequent and moderate/quite strong
- 3 points for each symptom that is continuous and significant/very strong or even disabling

SYMPTOMS	POINTS
STOMACH (Maximum 27) - Constipation - Diarrhoea - Irritable bowel syndrome - Stomach distension - Bloating especially after eating - Two sets of clothes needed for pre and post eating - Indigestion - Gas - Heartburn	1 2 2 3 2 3 3 2 18
HEAD (Maximum 24) - Headaches - Dizziness - Earaches - Blurred vision - Flushed cheeks - Feeling of 'sleepwalking' - Feeling unreal - Feeling 'spaced out'	2 2 3 3 10
WOMEN: (Maximum 24) - PMT - Water retention - Irregular menstruation - Painful breasts - Vaginal discharge - Vaginal itchiness - Thrush - Cystitis	3 2 2 7
BLOOD GLUCOSE: (Maximum 36) - Hungry between meals - Irritable or moody before meals - Shaky when hungry - Faintness when food is not eaten - Irregular pulse before and after eating - Headaches late morning - Waking in the early hours and not being able to get back to sleep - Abnormal cravings for sweet foods, bread, alcohol or caffeine	2 3 3 3 2 3 16

5 1

- Eating sweets increases hunger - Excessive appetite - Instant sugar 'high' followed by fatigue - Chilly feeling after eating	
MENTAL: (Maximum 30) - Anxiety - Depression - Irritability - Lethargy - Memory problems - Loss of concentration - Moodiness - Nightmares - Mental 'sluggishness' - *"Get up and go"* has got up and gone	
OTHER : (Maximum 72) - Food Intolerance - Dramatic fluctuations in weight from one day to the next - Poor circulation - Hands and feet sensitive to cold - Exhaustion - Feeling of being unable to cope - Constant fatigue - Muscle aches - Susceptibility to infection - Gasping for breath - Sighing often – 'hunger for air' - Tightness in chest - Chest aches - Cramps - Yawning easily - Insomnia - Excessive thirst - Easy weight gain - Coated tongue - Dry skin - Hair loss - Symptoms worse after consuming yeasty or sugary foods - Symptoms worse on damp, humid or rainy days - Athletes foot, dandruff or other fungal infection	

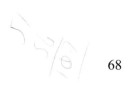

Again – the more points scored, and the more sections the points were scored in, the more likely it is that Candida is a problem for you. If you scored more than 50 points and scored in three or more sections it very likely that you are suffering from Candida.

How does Candida contribute to food cravings/addiction?

Candida is a living organism and every living thing has a natural self-preservation mechanism – we all fight to survive. The yeast living inside us is no exception. The Candida needs refined carbohydrates to feed it. It thrives on a weak immune system. It hates garlic and nutrients as they attack it and kill it off.

If you have Candida, you are having a constant battle with your body – you are trying to feel well but the Candida is trying to survive. The things needed for your well-being and the Candida's well-being are the opposite. When Candida really takes hold you will crave the foods that feed the yeast to ensure it grows and flourishes. If you crave burgers, you may well be craving the ketchup you put on them or the sugar, breadcrumbs and preservatives added to the meat. If you crave salad, it may well be the dressing that you are really after with its vinegar and sugar ingredients. You can pretty much guarantee you are not craving naked lettuce leaves and plain grilled meat.

You crave the items that feed the yeast, therefore, – all sugary foods, refined carbohydrates, concentrated fruit sugar, yeast and yeast derivatives and vinegary/pickled foods. There is evidence to suggest that eating yeast itself does not feed the yeast, but the consumption of bread and other foods containing yeast generally maintains the environment that the yeast needs to thrive in your body.

There are some great case studies from books on Candida, which give specific examples of the food cravings that Candida sufferers experience. Shirley S Lorenzani writes in her excellent book *"Candida – a Twentieth Century Disease"* about Candida driven cravings.

"Every night, at approximately 2am, Dr Jones dragged himself from bed, pulled on a pair of slacks over his pyjamas, and sped to an all-night grocery store. Roaming the aisles like a madman, he threw éclairs, pickles, smoked fish, and ice-cream into the cart. Unable to wait to feast at the kitchen table, he spread the items on the car seat, tore into a couple of wrappers, and began an engorgement that would end when the food did.

Candida overgrowth brings a craving for most of these forbidden (on the anti-Candida diet) foods – not just a preference but a strong virtually insatiable craving. People report dragging themselves out of bed at 2am to go to the all-night grocery."

Shirley S Lorenzani *"Candida – a Twentieth Century Disease"*

Another excellent book about Candida called *"The Yeast Syndrome"* is by John Parks Trowbridge and Morton Walker. There is a passage in this book about one of their patients:

"For a long time the woman had suffered with anorexia and bulimia. She dropped from 170 to 140 pounds... her menstrual flow stopped completely when food bingeing alternating with forced vomiting brought her weight down to 115 pounds... constant fatigue and addictive food cravings were additional troubles for Mrs. Bennett...Mrs. Bennett described several weeks of intense sugar cravings that had caused her to gobble down many refined carbohydrates – candy, cake, bread... " John Parks Trowbridge & Morton Walker *"The Yeast Syndrome."*

There are many other references in magazine articles, web pages and books on Candida. It is an absolutely documented fact that people with Candida overgrowth experience addict-like food cravings. People will drive to a grocery store in the middle of the night to feed the cravings and in so doing they will feed the yeast driving the cravings and make the cravings even worse in the future. The more you give into the cravings, the worse the Candida will get and the worse the cravings will get. It really is a vicious circle. The good news is that there is a virtuous circle, which is just as easy to get into, if you can break the vicious circle. The virtuous circle goes something like – you don't give into the cravings, you fight the yeast with diet and supplements, the cravings get easier, you get stronger, the Candida gets weaker, the cravings get easier and so on. The more you give into Candida induced cravings the worse they will get – you have to break the cycle and free yourself from the food addiction that is ruining your desire to be slim and probably your overall health and life.

How can you treat Candida?

There are some excellent writers who have focused on Candida such as Leon Chaitow, John Parks Trowbridge & Morton Walker and William G. Crook. There are three main pieces of advice for people suffering from Candida:
1) Starve the Candida overgrowth with diet.
2) Attack the Candida overgrowth with supplements that kill the yeast.
3) Treat the causes so that it doesn't come back.

1) **Starve the Candida.** The dietary advice varies a little but there is a basic diet that all practitioners would advocate – beautifully summed up by Trowbridge & Walker's expression MEVY – Meat/fish, Eggs, Vegetables and Natural Live Yoghurt (NLY). Then the authors vary a

70

little on what other things they allow on top of this. I have tried to summarise the advice from their books in the following table.

	THE YEAST SYNDROME Trowbridge & Walker	CANDIDA ALBICANS Chaitow	THE YEAST CONNECTION Crook
Protein	Meat, fish, eggs, tofu	Meat, fish, eggs, tofu	Meat, fish, eggs, tofu
Vegetables	All veg. & salad except: potatoes, sweet corn, beans, lentils, mushrooms	All veg. & salad except: potatoes, beans, pulses, lentils, chickpeas, mushrooms	All veg. & salad except mushrooms. (Eat potatoes, beans, sweet corn, squash, peas, beans cautiously)
Fruit	None	None for 2-3 weeks	None for 2-3 weeks
Dairy	NLY	NLY	NLY
Grains	None in the first few weeks. Corn, rice & quinoa in the 2nd stage. Oats, rye & wheat in stage 3	Brown Rice Millet Oats Quinoa Whole-wheat bread with no yeast	Barley, corn, millet, oats, rice, wheat (eat cautiously)
Other	Herbal tea	Herbal tea Nuts in shells Seeds Olive oil	Nuts Seeds Some oils
Key to avoid	Vinegar, mushrooms, yeast, sugar, refined carbohydrates	Vinegar, mushrooms, yeast, sugar, refined carbs, soy sauce, citric acid, MSG, all cheese including cottage, nuts not in shells	Vinegar, mushrooms, yeast, sugar, refined carbs, cheeses, melons, dried fruits
Re-introduction of foods	In 4 stages. Some grains in stage 2, most fruits, mushrooms & milk in stage 4	Stay off melons, mushrooms, cheese, milk, bread, vinegar as long as possible	All fruit in moderation, whole grains after a few weeks

2) **Attack the Candida** overgrowth with supplements that kill the yeast. Candida hates all of the following:

- Garlic – scientists have shown that garlic added to colonies of bacteria have ceased the functioning of that bacteria in minutes. Hence garlic is a well-known and well-documented antibacterial agent. Garlic has also been shown to be active against yeast and fungi.

- Biotin – research has shown that where a biotin deficiency exists, Candida changes more rapidly from its relatively harmless yeast form to its more dangerous multiplying form. Hence biotin has been shown to be a most useful vitamin in controlling Candida overgrowth.

- Olive oil – contains oleic acid, which prohibits the growth of the yeast in much the same way as biotin.

- Caprylic acid – which comes from coconut oil. You can get user friendly versions of this from some health food shops or from Internet suppliers.

- Lactobacillus Acidophilus – this is one of the major 'friendly' bacteria in our digestive systems and it can, therefore, be used to redress the balance of the gut flora and to fight off the Candida. Again health food shops and Internet suppliers will have this.

3) **Treat the cause** so that it doesn't return. Go back to the 'What causes Candida overgrowth?' section and see where the roots for your problem were:

- A weakened immune system – eat well, drink plenty of water, exercise regularly, don't smoke, drink alcohol in moderation, take time out to do things you enjoy, laugh, socialise, strive for balance. We all know the many things we can do to keep our health optimal and our immune system the strongest it can be.

- Over-consumption of refined carbohydrates – don't go back to consuming lots of sugary, yeasty, vinegary foods once you have got Candida back under control or you will be asking for it to return.

- Medication – steroids, antibiotics, birth control pills, hormones – try to avoid taking any of these if at all possible. Clearly serious illness requires treatment and unwanted pregnancies are not to be risked, but try to minimise the ingestion of all of the above. Is there an alternative form of contraception? See if you can heal a mild infection with Vitamin C and natural remedies before reaching for the antibiotics etc.

- Diabetes – you can still do things to help your situation if diabetes is the factor that has caused your yeast overgrowth. You can eat as healthy a diet as possible and thereby reduce the level of glucose in your blood, which may cause yeast overgrowth. Some individuals have been able to reduce the level of insulin they take and some even come off it altogether by following eating plans with little or no refined carbohydrates. If you are insulin dependent you must work with your doctor to work out the best eating plan and level of insulin for you. One thing that you can be sure of is that your health can only improve with the elimination of refined carbohydrates from your diet.
- Nutritional deficiency – eat as wide a variety as possible of vegetables, protein, whole grains, pulses and fruits and you should have no problem with nutritional deficiency. The most common causes of nutritional deficiency in the developed world are self inflicted – smoking, drinking too much alcohol, dieting and eating refined carbohydrates, leaving little room for more nutritious foods.

What else can I read if I want to know more?

"Candida – a Twentieth Century Disease" by Shirley Lorenzani (1986)
"The Yeast Syndrome" by John Parks Trowbridge MD and Morton Walker D.P.M. (1986)
"Candida Albicans – Could Yeast be your problem?" by Leon Chaitow (1987)
"The Yeast Connection" by William G. Crook MD (1983)
"The Complete Candida Yeast Guidebook" by Martin & Rona (2000)
"Beat Candida" by Gill Jacobs (1990)

Top tips for inspiration

This is worse than Star Wars! There is a parasite inside you, which is demanding to be fed, leading to you feeling dreadful – overweight, spaced out, tired, bloated and hardly able to get through the day. This parasite thrives on sugar, vinegary foods and yeast, as anyone who makes beer or wine will know. The more you feed it, the stronger it gets and the weaker you get.

This is war! Don't give this parasite anything it wants. Starve it by depriving it of all the foods it wants and kill it with supplements that it hates. How dare this thing try to take over your body? The good news is that you can devastate it very quickly in the battle. After just five days on a strict anti-Candida diet you can do a whole heap of damage. You

73

will have cravings like you have never known, in the early stages, and you could experience some quite unpleasant 'die-off' symptoms as you kill the yeast but this should only serve to strengthen your resolve. You may feel temporarily worse but soon you will start feeling quite dramatically better. Even after these first five tough days you could be feeling more energetic, less spaced out, the cravings should have subsided substantially and you will have lost pounds in weight.

Just imagine that every time you put a refined carbohydrate or vinegary food in your mouth you are putting petrol into the Candida's tank – you are literally fuelling this parasite that is making your life a misery. Keep this image in your mind every time you have a craving and you will soon rather do anything than feed this monster. Don't see refined carbohydrates as delicious – they are petrol for the enemy. Just visualise bacteria multiplying in your body with every mouthful you eat and this should ease the cravings.

If you don't attack this parasite it will just get stronger and stronger and you will feel weaker and weaker. You have to get it back in control sometime so start straight away before it gets any worse. Think of an end to tiredness and cravings. Think of an end to stomach bloating and digestive problems. Think of this horrible thing in your body and go for it.

KEY POINTS FROM CHAPTER 9

- Candida is a yeast that exists in all of us. It serves no useful purpose. When it gets out of control it can wreak havoc in our bodies.
- The main causes of Candida are 1) a weakened immune system, 2) over-consumption of refined carbohydrates, 3) medication, such as antibiotics and steroids, 4) diabetes and 5) nutritional deficiency.
- A wide variety of symptoms – physical and psychological – can indicate that Candida is overgrown inside you.
- Candida contributes to food cravings by demanding that you feed it – it loves refined carbohydrates, yeast and sugar in particular. This parasite can produce uncontrollable food cravings as it drives you to feed it so it can grow more and produce even stronger food cravings.
- You can treat it with a 3 step approach – 1) starve the Candida with your diet 2) attack the Candida overgrowth with supplements like garlic and 3) treat the causes so that it doesn't come back.
- This is war! You have to kill off this parasite before it does any more harm inside your body.

10

ONE PERSON'S POISON

Food Intolerance – everything you need to know

What is Food Intolerance?

The dictionary definition of 'allergy' is:
"The condition of reacting adversely to certain substances – especially food or pollen."

We should make the distinction at the outset that we are talking about Food Intolerance and not allergy as defined above. Food allergy refers to potential fatal reactions to a substance, such as with nut allergies. If someone has a food allergy the chances are that they were born with this allergy, will always have this allergy and it is a very serious condition. Common allergenic foods include nuts, shellfish, strawberries, I even know someone violently allergic to kiwis. If a person is exposed to the food, to which they are allergic, reactions range from breaking out into a rash, to extreme vomiting/stomach upset, or even death. We have all read tragic cases where people with an extreme allergy have died from being exposed to the food to which they are allergic. The sensitivity is extraordinary – my cousin discovered her young child had a nut allergy when she kissed him on the cheek hours after she had eaten a Chinese meal that contained peanut oil. The boy reacted to the minute trace of oil in the kiss on his cheek!

This chapter is not about **food allergy**. We are interested in **Food Intolerance**, which more generally means having an intolerance to a particular food or foods. By intolerance we mean an adverse reaction – not an extreme life threatening reaction as with food allergy – but any adverse reaction, which causes the person discomfort. Adverse reactions can include anything from gastrointestinal disorders to headaches and reactions which affect the mental state of the person who has consumed the food.

The following are the most common features of Food Intolerance (the what, when and how):

What – Food Intolerance develops with repeated overexposure to a particular food. The key words here are 'repeated' and 'overexposure'. It is common for people to become intolerant to foods that they eat a lot of and on a regular basis.

The foods most likely to cause intolerance are, therefore, the ones that are most common. The book "*The False Fat Diet*", by Elson M Haas MD & Cameron Stauth, which was written in the United States, says that the most common foods to cause sensitivity are:

1) Dairy products
2) Wheat
3) Corn *
4) Eggs
5) Soy *
6) Peanuts *
7) Sugar
* Corn, Soy and Peanuts are eaten very frequently in the US but far less so in the UK.

In Australia the most common Food Intolerances are to milk and wheat. Dr Brostoff, one of the leading Food Intolerance specialists in the UK, lists the most common foods causing intolerance in the UK as milk and wheat. Dr Brostoff also noted that for a doctor working in Taiwan, rice and soya beans were the chief culprits. The finger should point at whichever foods are most commonly eaten in the local cuisine.

When – Food Intolerance is not fixed as with food allergy and it can vary over time. People can find themselves susceptible to certain foods at different stages of their lives. For example, someone suffering from stress can develop intolerance to a food that they are consuming a lot of at the time and then be able to eat the food again in moderation at other times in their life. Pregnant women sometimes develop a sensitivity to a particular food that disappears after childbirth. My mother, for example, developed a marked sensitivity to the drink "Babycham", of all things, during her pregnancy!

The other interesting aspect of Food Intolerance, related to time, is that the adverse reaction is not immediate as with food allergy. For example, a person can eat a food to which they are intolerant and develop symptoms over the next twenty-four to forty-eight hours. When I had a wheat intolerance, I used to develop an upset stomach within hours and then the day after I felt completely exhausted and my muscles ached, as if I had run a marathon. This makes the identification of Food Intolerance all the more difficult as often many other foods have been eaten since the offending food, so it is difficult to pin-point the exact food, or foods, which have caused the reaction.

How – The offending food produces a state of well-being ranging from a slight mood change to an almost manic state of euphoria. This is when the addictive aspect of Food Intolerance takes hold. Gradually more and more of the offending food is needed to produce the state of well-being previously provided by a normal portion of the food. At this stage necessity is starting to replace desire. There is a need for the food and withdrawal symptoms will arise if the food is not eaten. For example, if you find that you get a headache mid-morning, if you don't have your usual breakfast, there may well be something that you are consuming at breakfast to which you have become intolerant.

What causes Food Intolerance?

The clue is in the text above – 'repeated' and 'overexposure'. It is estimated that we rely on as few as a dozen foods on a daily basis and that almost all of these will come from the milk, sugar and wheat food families. We eat toast or cereal for breakfast with milk (milk, sugar & wheat). We often have sugary snacks, and milk in tea and coffee, throughout the day (milk, sugar & wheat). We may have pasta, sandwiches or pizza for main meals (wheat and often milk and sugar again). If we have a salad, meat or fish, we may well have wheat or dairy with it, such as cheese, bread or crisp breads and so on. With repeated overexposure to any food, our bodies can become intolerant to this food and we will start to experience withdrawal symptoms if we don't have the food (this is when we are officially addicted to the food and the cravings for the food will be making us overeat).

There are other things that happen to make us more susceptible to Food Intolerance. Illness and medication can lead to a weakened immune system that will make us more susceptible to Food Intolerance and then this in turn weakens our immune system further (we are in the vicious circle downwards at this stage). Counting calories can also lead to Food Intolerance for a couple of reasons:

- We can weaken our immune system by taking in less fuel than we need.
- We tend to eat a restricted variety of foods when we count calories – we tend to eat more fruit, salad and other low calories foods and cut out steak, full fat dairy products and other high calorie foods. As we restrict the variety of foods that we eat, sticking to our favourites that

fill us up as much as possible for as few calories as possible, we are starting down the slippery slope towards Food Intolerance.

How do you know if you are affected by Food Intolerance?

As with Candida the range of symptoms related to Food Intolerance are many and varied. There are also remarkable overlaps, which is why, so often, people with extreme cravings and weight problems are suffering from both conditions. The complaints include:

Stomach – constipation; diarrhoea; irritable bowel syndrome; stomach distension; bloating, especially after eating; two sets of clothes needed for pre and post eating; indigestion; gas; heartburn.

Head – headaches; dizziness; flushed cheeks; feeling of 'sleepwalking'; feeling unreal; feeling 'spaced out'.

Women – PMT; water retention; irregular menstruation.

Blood Glucose – hungry between meals; irritable or moody before meals; shaky when hungry; faintness when food is not eaten; irregular pulse before and after eating; headaches late morning; waking in the early hours and not being able to get back to sleep; abnormal cravings for sweets or caffeine; eating sweets increases hunger; excessive appetite; instant sugar 'high' followed by fatigue; chilly feeling after eating.

Mental – anxiety; depression; irritability; lethargy; memory problems; loss of concentration; moodiness; nightmares; mental 'sluggishness'; reduced 'get up and go'.

Other – Food Intolerance; dramatic fluctuations in weight from one day to the next; exhaustion; feeling of being unable to cope; constant fatigue; muscle aches; susceptibility to infection; gasping for breath; sighing often – 'hunger for air'; chest aches; cramps; excessive thirst; easy weight gain; coated tongue; dry skin; itchiness/rashes.

Dr Brostoff uses a nice phrase which is "*thick note syndrome.*" Where doctors see a medical file which is thick and full of varied and seemingly unconnected complaints, they would be well advised to ask the person what they are eating.

How does Food Intolerance contribute to food cravings/addiction?

The real irony is that the foods to which you are intolerant are the foods that you crave. Just as the drug addict or smoker craves their fix, so you crave the substances that are causing you harm. It starts off with a particular food or drink that you consume on regular occasions. The most common offenders are dairy products and wheat as we have them in so many different forms during the day. Any substance that we eat daily can start to cause problems and those we eat regularly, several times a day, are the chief suspects. It takes three to four days for a digested substance to pass through our bodies, so we can overload our bodies with one particular substance if we eat it daily or even more often.

Our bodies then literally become 'intolerant' to the food – i.e. they can't cope with any more of it. You would think that we would shun a food if we had become intolerant to it but in fact the addiction that goes with Food Intolerance actually means that the opposite happens. If we remember back to the definition of addiction, we go through these stages with Food Intolerance:

- We start with an uncontrollable craving.
- We then need more and more of the offending substance in order to get the same 'high'.
- We develop physical and/or psychological dependence.
- We suffer the adverse effects.

I developed a bizarre intolerance to cocoa which resulted from over-consumption of the delicious milky coffees that I experienced when I first came across *Starbucks*. I found myself craving 'grande decaf lattes' to such an extent that I could easily drink four or five a day. This gave me around three pints of milk per day but ironically it was the cocoa dusting on the top that I was really craving. I found myself needing more and more each day and, if I didn't get my fix, I would get quite anxious and irritable. I realised it was the cocoa, and not the coffee or the milk, when one day there was no cocoa powder available and I realised that the froth without the powder on top did nothing to satisfy my needs. I would have an instant and significant 'high' as soon as I tasted the powder and serious withdrawal symptoms if I went without it for even a few hours.

If you want to know what you are intolerant to, simply ask yourself honestly the food(s) you would least like to give up. If you cannot imagine life without bread or cereal you should suspect wheat. If you can't face a day without eggs in any form (e.g. some pasta is egg based) then eggs could be your problem. It is so cruel but the foods that we

79

don't crave – those we could take or leave – are the foods that we need to keep in our diets. However, even these we need to eat in moderation and irregularly as anything can become a problem if we have repeated overexposure.

The following extracts from books on Food Intolerance capture the addictive nature of Food Intolerance beautifully:

"Specific allergic adaptation to foods and chemicals is an addiction as devastating as addiction to tobacco or drugs. In my opinion, only heroin or morphine addiction are more potent and destructive than severe food addiction, which I would put on a par with alcoholism."
Dr Richard Mackarness *"Not all in the mind"*

"Bread is another good example of an addictive allergy. Some individuals just cannot go without bread, even for a day – toast for breakfast, sandwiches for lunch, bread for dinner. The standard reaction to the suggestion of 'no more bread' is the statement 'what is there left to eat?'. This type of person can quite easily consume up to one loaf of bread a day and it is usual to find them consuming half a loaf."
"These addictive foods are always over-consumed and at frequent intervals. If you miss eating them you will start to feel bad. When you miss having your regular fix you start to have withdrawal symptoms just like a drug addict. Your body starts rebelling against the removal of the food on which it has come to depend."
Robert Buist *"Food Intolerance"*

"...we reach a stage of addiction : the patient craves the food and wants to eat it often, even to binge the food. The reason is that by this stage, ironically, the patient gets the symptoms only if he or she doesn't eat the food."
Dr Keith Mumby *"The Allergy Handbook"*

"Food addiction differs only in degree of severity from a drug addiction."
"The American humorist Don Marquis once said that 'ours is a world where people don't know what they want and are willing to go through hell to get it.' This is a good description of the food addict, who doesn't know the exact nature of the food he craves, but is willing to eat compulsively, to the point of addiction, in order to get it."
In reference to a clinic patient: "I've reached the point where I am afraid to eat any longer. Once I start eating, I feel as if I simply cannot stop."

Discussing a food addict: "He may wake up in the middle of the night and help himself to more food. Sometimes family members will joke that he seems to be addicted to sweets, cheese, steak, or whatever is his favourite treat. If only they knew how right they are!"
Theron Randolph & Ralph Moss *"Allergies – Your Hidden Enemy."*

"Millions of men, women and children suffer from the addictive form of food allergy... Obese people are living testaments to the strength of food addiction... The foods to which the compulsive eater has an addictive allergy are never skipped, and eating for the relief of food-related withdrawal symptoms may become the obese person's interest in life... Progressive overweight develops as the advancing stage of allergic food addiction requires increasing doses of the specific food(s) to satisfy the craving... the compulsive eater is not overwhelmed with emotional problems or an unfulfilled need for love that requires oral gratification. He is a chronic foodaholic with a serious but easily diagnosable nonpsychological ailment."
Dr Marshall Mandell & Lynne Scanlon *"5-Day Allergy Relief System"*

"Food reactions are the single most common cause of the cravings that destroy diets. These cravings, which are far harder to resist than mere hunger, are similar to the physical urges experienced by alcoholics or cigarette smokers."
Elson M Haas MD & Cameron Stauth *"The False Fat Diet"*

All of these passages confirm why you overeat – when all you want is to be slim. One of the reasons is almost certainly that you are intolerant to some foods. The intolerance will drive addict-like cravings, which is why you feel you have no control over your eating whatsoever.

How can you treat Food Intolerance?

To regain control you need to identify those foods to which you are intolerant and eliminate them from your diet. You will go through intense withdrawal symptoms while you do this but the good news is that these should last fewer than five days – just a bit more than the time it takes for a substance to pass through your body completely. You will then find that, if you eat the offending food after avoiding it for some time, you may experience extreme and sudden reactions, which is your body's way of confirming that this food is not good for you.

The key steps to treating Food Intolerance are, therefore, quite simple – find out what is causing you problems and stop eating it. Don't get depressed thinking you are about to give up some foods for life. Unlike food allergy, which remains for a life-time, Food Intolerance does come and go over time. Hence you could find yourself intolerant to, say, dairy products, during a stressful period of your life when your immune system is particularly low and you may find you can tolerate dairy products again when your health is better. Many people find that they can re-introduce foods to which they have been intolerant in time, when their immunity has recovered, but only on an infrequent basis. In other words, you will probably find that you can return to consuming any food or drink, in time, but you are likely to find that your symptoms and cravings reappear quite quickly as soon as you eat the substance too much or too often.

Step 1 – Identify the Foods

You can identify the foods to which you are intolerant in two main ways:
1) You can find a nutritionist or Food Intolerance practitioner to help you.
2) You can find out yourself with a bit of 'trial and error'.

1) Nutritionists and Food Intolerance practitioners use a number of ways to identify Food Intolerance. Some will just ask you to keep a food diary and then ask you questions in much the same way as the 'trial and error' method. Some will start with the most common food intolerances and eliminate these from your diet to see how you get on. Some will do skin tests or blood tests or analyse your hair, skin and nails for signs of problems. A quite common method of diagnosis involves testing strength and pressure points by placing suspect foods on your energy lines throughout your body. An offending food placed on the energy lines will significantly impact your strength and a food that you are fine with does not. All I can suggest is for you to be open minded to whichever method your practitioner uses – they do know what they are doing.

2) With the trial and error method there are a number of things that you can try:
   - The best rule of thumb is always that the foods that you crave are the ones that are most likely to be causing you problems. Anything that you eat often and in large, or increasing, quantities should be suspected. Anything that you really can't imagine **not** eating is your offending food.
   - You absolutely must start a food diary as changes can be subtle over time and it may be that you need to compare diary entries days or weeks apart to notice how far you have progressed. However, the outcome could also be quite dramatic and not at

all subtle. Buy a notebook and write down everything you eat and how you feel afterwards. This alone may establish a pattern. For example, if after every entry with bread, pasta, cakes or biscuits you record that you experience bloating and stomach problems, you can start to suspect wheat as a problem.

- When you have started recording what you eat and how it makes you feel you can try to cut out the foods that you suspect and again there are a number of ways in which you can do this. You can keep your eating patterns as close to your normal eating as possible and just cut out foods that you suspect or, at the other extreme, you can start a very limited diet and re-introduce foods from there. This is when we move onto Step 2:

Step 2 – Stop eating them!

When you move onto food elimination it is really important to keep that food diary going to notice any changes that do occur. There are a number of different options that you can try. We will list them in order of the easiest to follow. However, please note that the easiest to follow may not necessarily deliver the best results:

- The easiest option is to keep eating mostly the same foods – just cut out a few of the main foods that you suspect are causing you problems. This has the advantage of having a minimal impact on your eating habits but it is unlikely to identify all the problem foods and it may take a long time to get results.

- The next easiest option is to cut out the most common Food Intolerances (wheat, dairy, eggs, corn, soy, peanuts, sugar etc). This will be more likely to eliminate some of your problem foods but it may also mean that you avoid some foods unnecessarily as they may not be a problem for you.

- The option I strongly recommend is to do the 5 day kick-start eating plan in this book. This eliminates all refined carbohydrates and any foods that you suspect are causing you problems. This will give you quick results with cravings and weight loss and it is short enough a period to stick to. It will eliminate your problem foods and you can then re-introduce these, one at a time, after the five days to see how you feel. Keeping a comprehensive food diary, after every new food is re-introduced, will be all that you need to confirm the problem foods for you.

- The most extreme measure ever suggested in books on Food Intolerance is to go on what is called a 'lamb and pears' elimination diet. This literally means eating nothing but lamb and pears for five days. I do not advise this a) because it is not good for vegetarians and b) because it is unnecessarily extreme. You don't need to go this far to identify and give up your offending foods.

There are two ways in which the avoidance of foods can help identify and, therefore, treat Food Intolerance. It may sound simple and obvious but when you stop eating a problem food you should feel better and when you start eating a problem food again you should feel worse. The slight complication is that **initially**, when you first stop eating an offending food, you may feel a lot worse and your cravings could be as bad as ever. Remember you are craving food because you are trying to avoid the withdrawal symptoms that you get when you don't have the food to which you are intolerant. Hence, when you first stop eating the problem food, the withdrawal symptoms are going to come out in force. This is where the food diary will really help as you may record feeling exhausted, lethargic and depressed and with unbearable cravings for one to five days. However, after these first few days you should feel much better. If you avoid an offending food for a few days or weeks and then go back to eating it you can suffer quite dramatic bad symptoms. However, if you avoid an offending food for a long period of time, such as months or years, you could equally find that you have no problems with the food that previously caused you trouble.

Food Intolerance is quite a complex and sensitive area and it reflects your overall well-being at any one time, so it will change as you do. A food diary will really help to show what causes immediate problems (e.g. cravings, bloating) and what causes problems up to a day after (stomach upset, fatigue). You need to become highly tuned in to what you eat and how it makes you feel.

Other tips for the 'trial and error' method include:

- eat single foods not processed foods. If you react badly to a cake, you won't know if sugar, wheat, eggs or dairy products are your problem as they are all in a cake. To test each substance you need to eat it on its own, e.g. to test wheat, eat shredded wheat (100% whole-wheat) on its own; to test dairy products, try milk on its own; to test eggs, eat eggs on their own etc.

- eat one food at a time – one of the best ways to test foods is to avoid them for at least five days (so that there are no traces of them in your system) and then re-introduce them one by one and check for symptoms. e.g. have wheat on its own for breakfast, have only eggs for lunch and then only corn for dinner. As this is very restrictive it can be made easier by mixing one food to be tested with foods that you know don't cause you a problem. It is rare for people to be intolerant to meat, fish and vegetables so have these at each meal with just one other food that you are testing at that meal. If you suffer symptoms, you can then be pretty sure which food has caused the problems.

- eat food a few hours apart – don't test one food within four hours of another as the symptoms may take time to show and you could mistakenly think the second food has caused the problem.

- assume the foods you most crave and would most miss are the ones causing you problems. If there are any foods that you never crave, and could happily live without, sadly these are the ones that you need to have in your eating plan until your Food Intolerance is brought under control.

In summary, to treat Food Intolerance you need to identify the food(s) to which you are intolerant and eliminate them for as long as necessary. The complications are in the detail – how long is necessary? How do you know which foods? I hope the above section has suggested a number of ways in which you can identify your own problem foods, how you can cut them out of your diet and how you can re-introduce them to test them for confirmation. The final stage, once your immunity and health is restored, is to eat as wide a variety of food as possible, trying not to eat any food every day and keeping a lookout for any cravings and other symptoms which could indicate that Food Intolerance has returned.

What else can I read if I want to know more?

"*Food Intolerance – What it is & How to cope with it*" by Robert Buist (1984)
"*5-day Allergy Relief System*" by Dr Marshall Mandell and Lynne Scanlon (1979)
"*The Allergy Handbook*" by Dr Keith Mumby (1988)
"*Allergies – Your Hidden Enemy?*" by Theron Randolph MD & Ralph W. Moss PhD (1981)
"*Not all in the Mind*" by Dr Richard Mackarness (1976)
"*The False Fat Diet*" by Elson M Haas MD & Cameron Stauth (2001)
"*The Complete Guide to Food Allergy and Intolerance*" by Dr Jonathan Brostoff & Linda Gamlin (1989)

Top tips for inspiration

This is one of the easiest conditions to address. Unlike Candida, which can take weeks to get under control, you can stop the cravings which follow from Food Intolerance in a maximum of five days. It takes fewer than five days for the substance causing you problems to have totally cleared itself from your body and there will then be no reason for you to crave that substance any longer. You are likely to have tough withdrawal symptoms for the first few days, but then you will feel better than you have done for ages – mentally more alert, more energetic and clear headed.

Just think – you can be free from your Food Intolerance cravings in just five days. You can be rid of that puffy, red face that greets you each morning. You can be free from stomach bloating and digestive problems that are caused by intolerance to a particular food.

One of the best inspirational tips to get you going is that you could lose pounds as soon as you stop eating a food to which you are intolerant. Food Intolerance leads to dramatic water retention. When you stop eating a food that is causing you problems you are likely to lose pounds very quickly indeed and you will find that your rings, shoes and clothes fit better than ever before.

KEY POINTS FROM CHAPTER 10

- Food **allergy** is the condition of reacting badly to certain substances – like nuts or strawberries. It can be life threatening. It is not what this chapter is about.
- Food **Intolerance** is the condition of being intolerant to a particular food or foods. It is not life threatening but it can make you feel quite unwell in a variety of ways.
- The key cause of Food Intolerance is repeated overexposure to a certain food – having too much of it and too often.
- The symptoms of Food Intolerance are many and varied and include physical as well as psychological complaints.
- Food Intolerance leads to food cravings because you ironically crave the foods to which you are intolerant. In fact, a sure sign of Food Intolerance is having a substance that you crave uncontrollably and try to eat as often as possible.
- You treat Food Intolerance quite simply by not eating the foods to which you are intolerant. You probably won't have to avoid them for ever as, when your immune system is stronger, you may well be able to tolerate them again.

11

BLOOD GLUCOSE – TOO LOW OR TOO HIGH?

Hypoglycaemia – everything you need to know

What is Hypoglycaemia?

Hypoglycaemia is literally a Greek translation from "*hypo*" meaning 'under', "*glykis*" meaning 'sweet' and "*emia*" meaning 'in the blood together'. The three bits all put together mean low blood glucose. (It is sometimes known as hyperinsulinism as the opposite of low blood glucose is excessive insulin). It follows that the causes of Hypoglycaemia are the factors which trigger the pancreas to release insulin in response to a sudden rise in blood glucose level. Sugar and refined carbohydrates are the main offenders but caffeine, allergic substances, stress and alcohol may all prompt a similar response.

In 1924, during the investigation of diabetes and the development of insulin, it was observed by Dr Seale Harris that non-diabetic people had reactions similar to diabetics who had taken too much insulin. A paper on 'hyperinsulinism' was published in the Journal of the American Medical Association. Further research by Harris found that Hypoglycaemia, as the condition became known, was the result of a defect in the blood glucose regulating system. Subsequent research has shown how crucial the blood glucose balance is for a healthy body and mind and yet, eighty years after the initial studies, many doctors believe that millions of people are still undiagnosed as hypoglycaemic. Instead they are labelled neurotic, anxious, depressed, fatigued, stressed, anti-social and moody. They may also be labelled alcoholic or bulimic if they suffer from compulsive drinking and eating, as many hypoglycaemics do.

If a diabetic takes too much insulin the following symptoms may arise – weakness, tremors, clammy hands, sweating, fainting, blackouts, hunger, thirst, mental confusion, exhaustion, irritability and many other symptoms. As the brain and central nervous system rely on stable and adequate supplies of blood glucose for normal function, the most dramatic symptoms of Hypoglycaemia are shown in the emotional and mental state of a person. Many, if not all, psychiatric disorders can be prompted by low blood glucose – amnesia, negativism, personality changes, maniacal behaviour, emotional instability and delirium.

Diabetics who have their insulin injection and then delay their meal, or eat too little relative to the amount of insulin injected, can display quite alarming symptoms. In the extreme they can lapse into a coma and die.

I have witnessed a diabetic in a state of low blood glucose after taking too much insulin relative to food intake one evening. He had a total lack of awareness and co-ordination to the extent that, when his girlfriend suggested that he should put his shoes on, he just nodded 'yes' and didn't move. The request was repeated on several occasions until those around him realised that he could not register what his shoes were, let alone whether or not he had them on, and how to put them on if they were not already on! He was extremely withdrawn, distant and completely dopey. (Incidentally this diabetic was a twenty-six year old Cambridge graduate). The apathetic confused disorientated 'overeater' who sits for hours staring at the floor or ceiling after a binge may be suffering from similar problems with blood glucose.

In a non-diabetic person, as food is eaten, the pancreas releases insulin to compensate for the rise in blood glucose which occurs as food is ingested. (If this process did not occur the person would be diabetic). Diabetes is initially diagnosed by the presence of sugar in the urine and then a blood test is taken for confirmation. Thus the role of the pancreas is to ensure that sugar balance is maintained with no sugar leaving the body as a waste product.

The function performed by the pancreas is probably the most delicate balancing operation performed by the body and there is increasing evidence that the modern western diet is disturbing this mechanism. From the caveperson era to the industrial revolution, the human diet featured meat, fish, vegetables, fruits and berries and then grains such as wheat and rice once they became available. The current consumption of cakes, sweets, biscuits, ice-cream, sugary drinks and so on is historically unprecedented. Furthermore, sugar is found in almost all modern consumer foods from cereal to yoghurt and from baked beans to prepared salads.

Medical opinion is divided on the subject of the prevalence of disturbed carbohydrate tolerance or 'Reactive Hypoglycaemia' as a result of the typical western diet. However, it cannot be disputed that blood glucose will remain more stable, and the pancreas will have to react less, on a diet of protein and vegetables than on a diet of sugar and refined carbohydrates. Given this undisputable fact and given the evidence we have of the impact of blood glucose level on the body and mind, it remains a complete mystery to me why so many doctors dismiss the notion of Hypoglycaemia and treat people with anti-depressants and other drugs before trying a change in diet.

On a diet of fat/protein and vegetables, blood glucose remains well balanced and quite stable whereas on a diet of sugar and refined carbohydrates the pancreas is overworked at regular intervals and the blood glucose level peaks and troughs with the amplitude of a wave frequency motion. If you had a very sophisticated pair of scales, capable of weighing individual grains of rice, would you put a sack of potatoes on them? This is what you are doing to your body if you eat refined carbohydrates at regular intervals and your tolerance for them is anything less than perfect.

Our bodies are used to animal and plant food and they have performed well on such a diet for thousands of years. Refined carbohydrates are foreign substances and not ones needed or welcomed by the body. The choice is yours. You can believe in Hypoglycaemia, even if many doctors remain too narrow-minded to accept it. Try the diet for Hypoglycaemia and if you don't feel **more** emotionally stable, physically refreshed and alert, and **less** anxious, depressed and frequently hungry then go back to your old eating habits. The deciding factor, if you presently overeat, will be if you don't lose weight and end the nightmare of continuous insatiable cravings on the eating plan for Hypoglycaemia, then return to your previous eating habits. I know that if you follow the eating plan for Candida, Food Intolerance and Hypoglycaemia your natural weight can be reached quickly and easily and you can be rid of addict-like cravings indefinitely.

If we apply the theory of Hypoglycaemia to eating disorders, consider the overeater who tries to starve for a day and becomes restless, crabby, irritable, depressed and sometimes emotionally unstable. The overeater then breaks their fast with, say, a confectionery bar and becomes hyperactive, manic, bubbly, talkative and alert for probably no more than two hours before the depression and emotional instability returns. The psychological theory suggests that the overeater is depressed and unstable during the fast because they are not blotting out emotional problems by eating. When they eat they feel temporary relief and then feel guilty afterwards. Undoubtedly the overeater does feel guilty after eating, but it may be low blood glucose causing the symptoms of depression and instability rather than fundamental psychological problems. This seems to have been overlooked by doctors and psychologists to date.

Recent research has shown that **fluctuations** in blood glucose are as important to Hypoglycaemia as the **actual** level of blood glucose. If the blood glucose level falls *rapidly* below normal, symptoms include sweating, weakness, hunger, rapid beating of the heart and a feeling of fear or anxiety. If the blood glucose level falls *slowly* over a period of time, a person may suffer headaches, blurred vision, mental confusion, crabbiness, irritability and incoherent speech. Then, if this fall is sustained for a period of hours, the symptoms may include outburst of temper, extreme depression, sleepiness, restlessness, negativism, emotional instability, manic behaviour and general personality disorders.

Consider this in the light of the overeater who starves and binges. As the fast starts, the blood glucose level falls slowly and the person becomes confused and unable to concentrate at work. Reactions slow down, memory and mechanical ability suffer and headaches may be extremely unpleasant ('hunger headaches'). The overeater then binges and their blood glucose level rises rapidly and then falls rapidly as insulin is released in compensation. This rapid fall in the blood glucose level prompts hunger, weakness and a feeling of profound anxiety. This may not be simply anxiety about having binged, but general anxiety caused by Hypoglycaemia.

What causes Hypoglycaemia?

The key cause of Hypoglycaemia is the consumption of refined carbohydrates. If you remember from Chapter 2, if you eat an apple your body normally releases the right amount of insulin to 'mop' up the glucose in your blood after eating the apple and to return your blood glucose level to normal. If it doesn't do this you are diabetic or your pancreas is not working properly due to the overload you have been placing on it with the food that you normally eat. If you drink a carton of apple juice, your body thinks you have eaten, say, twenty apples and releases the amount of insulin needed to cope with lots of apples. Because you haven't eaten twenty apples there is an excess of insulin in your body and this will have the effect of lowering your blood glucose level below normal. You are now in a state of Hypoglycaemia, by definition, as your blood glucose level is low.

Hence the state of Hypoglycaemia can be brought on temporarily and quickly by consuming refined carbohydrates. When we say that someone has Hypoglycaemia what we are really saying is that their pancreas/insulin releasing mechanism is out of balance and that they are constantly in a state of high or low blood glucose. They are rarely at a nice, even, steady level of blood glucose. They swing from one extreme to the other and suffer the energy highs and lows that go with it. This is almost certainly as a result of long term consumption of refined carbohydrates.

Some people do seem to be able to eat refined carbohydrates and 'get away with it'. Their bodies don't seem to release too much insulin, which suggests that some people may be more susceptible to Hypoglycaemia than others. However, in the majority of people, prolonged consumption of refined carbohydrates is likely to cause Hypoglycaemia. In some people it even leads to diabetes. Maturity onset diabetes is almost always preceded by Hypoglycaemia (often people did not know that they were suffering from Hypoglycaemia before they were diagnosed as diabetic). Some people's pancreases go from producing too much insulin to not producing enough, or any at all, which is the definition of diabetes.

Diabetes and Hypoglycaemia can both be greatly helped by following an eating plan which contains no refined carbohydrates whatsoever. Eating refined carbohydrates can be a cause of Hypoglycaemia and maturity onset diabetes.

How do you know if you are affected by Hypoglycaemia?

Hypoglycaemia can be diagnosed with a glucose tolerance test, which involves a series of blood tests being taken, after a glucose drink has been drunk, to measure the person's tolerance for sugar. This test is rarely performed at the suggestion of a doctor and it may be difficult to persuade your doctor to refer you for one. The perfectly acceptable alternative is to try the eating plan for Hypoglycaemia and keep a food diary to notice if your symptoms improve or disappear altogether.

If you follow a low carbohydrate diet for a period of time and your symptoms improve considerably you can be pretty certain that Hypoglycaemia has been a problem for you. One of the best tests, much more readily available than a glucose tolerance test, is to follow the Phase 1 eating plan in this book for five days. If you have stable energy levels, a clear head and your other symptoms of Hypoglycaemia have subsided then you can be sure that Hypoglycaemia was a problem for you.

The symptoms of Hypoglycaemia include the following:

Head – headaches; dizziness; blurred vision; feeling of 'sleepwalking'; feeling unreal; feeling 'spaced out'.

Women – PMT.

Blood Glucose – hungry between meals; irritable or moody before meals; shaky when hungry; faintness when food is not eaten; irregular pulse before and after eating; headaches late morning; waking in the early hours and not being able to get back to sleep; abnormal cravings for sweets or caffeine; eating sweets increases hunger; excessive appetite; instant sugar 'high' followed by fatigue; chilly feeling after eating.

Mental – anxiety; depression; irritability; lethargy; memory problems; loss of concentration; moodiness; nightmares; mental 'sluggishness'; *"get up and go"* has got up and gone.

Other – dramatic fluctuations in weight from one day to the next; exhaustion; feeling of being unable to cope; constant fatigue; excessive thirst; easy weight gain.

How does Hypoglycaemia contribute to food cravings/addiction?

This is a really simple one. As soon as your blood glucose level falls below normal your body will cry out for food. It will crave anything, but most likely sweet foods, to get your blood glucose level back up again. When your hands are shaking, you feel a bit sweaty, a bit light headed or even faint in extreme cases, this is your body begging you to eat. You reach for a confectionery bar and immediately feel better, almost euphoric, as your blood glucose level shoots up. However, this is another substance alien to your pancreas so your body overproduces insulin, your blood glucose level falls below normal again and the cravings continue.

This is exactly why once you start bingeing you can't stop – because your blood glucose level swings from high to below normal and as soon as it is below normal you cannot resist food so you eat and it shoots back up to high again. It is a vicious circle that so many of us go through several times a day.

How can you treat Hypoglycaemia?

This is pretty simple too – stop eating refined carbohydrates. You should switch to a low carbohydrate diet (the kick-start eating plan in Chapter 13 of this book) for a few days to confirm the diagnosis and to see just how well you can feel. Then continue to eat only **un**refined (whole-meal) carbohydrates.

Before insulin was discovered, even diabetics could survive by following a practically zero carbohydrate diet so that no insulin was needed by the body. Hypoglycaemia can be managed much more easily than this and you don't need to avoid all carbohydrates – just refined ones.

What else can I read if I want to know more?

"Hypoglycaemia – The Disease your Doctor Won't Treat" by Saunders & Ross (1980)
"Low Blood glucose (Hypoglycaemia) The twentieth century Epidemic?" by Martin L Budd (1983)
"New low blood sugar & you" by Carlton Fredericks (1985)

Top tips for inspiration

This condition is the most serious of all three. Candida can make you feel really ill but it is not life threatening. Food Intolerance, similarly, can make you feel most unwell but it is food **allergy** that is life threatening, not Food **Intolerance**. Hypoglycaemia is potentially very serious. It can lead to Diabetes, which is the fourth leading cause of death in most developed countries, third in the US. At the very least, Hypoglycaemia is your body's way of telling you that something is wrong. It is telling you that your pancreas cannot cope with what you are putting into your body and your pancreas is a vital organ for health and well-being.

If you care at all about your health, if the thought of possibly becoming diabetic and injecting insulin once or twice a day frightens you, then take this early warning very seriously.

You have got a highly sensitive balancing system in your body and you are ruining it day by day, hour by hour. You may as well take a set of laboratory scales, capable of weighing a feather, and throw a brick on them!

This is not just about weight – your whole health and body functions are at stake here. You simply must start being kind to your body by giving it foods to nourish it rather than bombarding it with junk.

KEY POINTS FROM CHAPTER 11

- Hypoglycaemia literally means low blood glucose.
- Hypoglycaemia is primarily caused by the over-consumption of refined carbohydrates. Some people appear to be more susceptible to it than others but the incidence of Hypoglycaemia is now believed to be very widespread.
- The symptoms of Hypoglycaemia are many and varied and include physical as well as psychological complaints.
- Hypoglycaemia leads to food cravings because when your blood glucose level falls below normal, as a result of too much insulin being released, your body will beg you to eat to raise your blood glucose level again. If you eat something else that will result in too much insulin being produced (a refined carbohydrate), your blood glucose level will fall below normal again and you will be in a vicious cycle of food craving.
- You treat Hypoglycaemia quite simply by not eating refined carbohydrates. Some people find that they need to limit all carbohydrates, until their insulin mechanism retunes, but invariably people can eat whole-meal carbohydrates safely.

12

COMPLETING THE JIGSAW

Candida, Food Intolerance and Hypoglycaemia and how overeating links with all of them

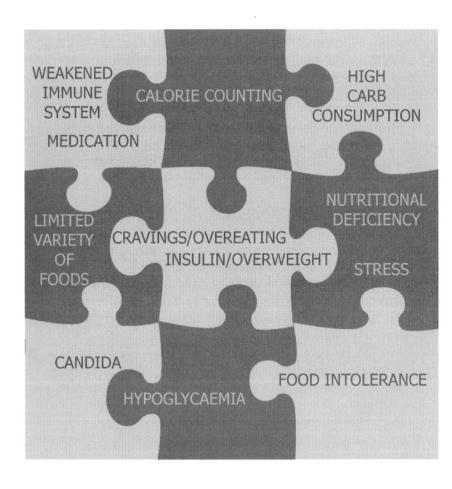

WEAKENED IMMUNE SYSTEM

MEDICATION

CALORIE COUNTING

HIGH CARB CONSUMPTION

LIMITED VARIETY OF FOODS

CRAVINGS/OVEREATING INSULIN/OVERWEIGHT

NUTRITIONAL DEFICIENCY

STRESS

CANDIDA

HYPOGLYCAEMIA

FOOD INTOLERANCE

If you have read lots about dieting, eating and health you may already have come across the conditions of Candida, Food Intolerance and Hypoglycaemia. You may well have read books that say eat carbohydrate not fat and others that say eat fat not carbohydrate. You are probably so confused that you don't know which way to turn.

This chapter pieces together all the bits of the jigsaw that you may have read about and makes sense of them. It explains causes and effects and why you may be suffering from any, or all, of the three conditions that can cause food cravings and overeating. The answer to the carbohydrate vs. fat debate is actually that you need both (which I'm sure you worked out long ago). You need carbohydrates but you don't need **refined** carbohydrates. You need fat but you don't need transunsaturated fat (manufactured fat). How and when you eat carbohydrate and fat will be explained in detail in Part 4.

For now we have the following pieces in the jigsaw and the following explanations for how they all fit together...

You overeat because of one thing that you are doing and three conditions that you may be suffering from. The one thing that you are doing is calorie counting and the three conditions are Candida, Food Intolerance and Hypoglycaemia. There are causes of all of these conditions so let us start piecing together what has caused the conditions and what the outcome has been:

CAUSES	CALORIE COUNTING MEDICATION STRESS WEAKENED IMMUNE SYSTEM HIGH CARB' CONSUMPTION LIMITED VARIETY OF FOODS

CONDITIONS	CANDIDA FOOD INTOLERANCE HYPOGLYCAEMIA

OUTCOMES	CRAVINGS OVEREATING OVER PRODUCTION OF INSULIN OVERWEIGHT

The causes shown in the top of the three boxes above are all those that we covered in Chapters 9 to 11 when we explored the conditions Candida, Food Intolerance and Hypoglycaemia. Remember how calorie counting leads to a limited variety of foods being consumed and how it leads to an increase in the consumption of carbohydrates as calorie counters cut back on fat and protein. We also discussed a weakened immune system (nutritional deficiency), medication (such as antibiotics and the pill) and stress as causes of each of the three conditions in this book. The outcomes of all of the conditions are food cravings, overeating, over production of insulin and overweight.

Trying to show this as a flow diagram is quite a challenge because almost every cause, condition and outcome are so interrelated. Don't worry too much about tracing every arrow. The key thing to take out of the flow diagram on the next page is just how interlinked the jigsaw pieces are.

The two way arrows show things that have causal links both ways. For example cravings can lead to Food Intolerance (because they can drive you to consuming just your 'favourite' foods) but also Food Intolerance leads to cravings as you crave the foods to which you are intolerant.

The one way arrows show things that have a one-way cause. For example calorie counting leads to a high consumption of carbohydrates (because people who count calories cut fat and protein down as a percentage of their food intake) but a high consumption of carbohydrates does not lead to calorie counting.

It is very likely that you are suffering from one, or all, of the conditions of Candida, Food Intolerance and Hypoglycaemia if you have been experiencing the extreme cravings that are known to sabotage the best of slimming intentions. It would not be surprising if you were suffering from more than one, as the overlaps and links between them are extraordinary.

The flow diagram shows the links between counting calories, medication, the stress of modern life, over-consumption of carbohydrates, a weakened immune system and a limited variety of foods. The diagram shows the causal links (i.e. what leads to what) between all of these factors. Any one of them can start the vicious circle and then the others join in. Please keep referring back to the diagram to see just how closely all of these conditions fit together. You are now piecing together the jigsaw that explains all the other things that you may have read about.

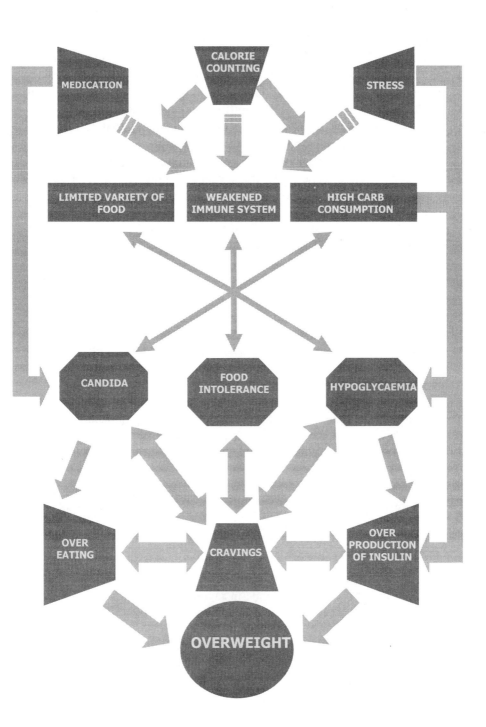

Calorie Counting

When we count calories we tend to restrict high fat foods and fill up on low calorie foods instead. Indeed almost all low calorie regimes tell the slimmer to avoid fat like the plague – no butter or spreads, no red meat, no cream, no real milk. Only low fat products are allowed – skimmed milk, fat free yoghurt, low fat muffins and manufacturers have even come up with low fat crisps and chips! Remember that low fat/low calorie foods are generally high in carbohydrate and high fat foods generally have no carbohydrate e.g. butter or steak. The staple foods of the calorie counter (especially female calorie counters) tend to be salads, fruits, crisp breads, and rice cakes – all of these are high in carbohydrate with almost no fat or protein whatsoever. When someone switches to a low calorie diet, and cuts out a lot of fat and protein, they have to fill up on carbohydrates, as these are the only things left.

As regards cravings, calorie counting leads to cravings both indirectly and directly:

- Calorie counting directly causes cravings because we become hungry having deprived our bodies of much needed sustenance. Our bodies respond to this by craving calories – any will do just to top up the energy deficit that we are experiencing. Hence calorie counting directly leads us to crave food.

- Indirectly calorie counting leads to a high consumption of carbohydrates, which fuels Candida, Food Intolerance and Hypoglycaemia and these in turn lead to cravings.

- Calorie counting leads to a weakened immune system as we quite literally take in less fuel than we need to sustain ourselves and our bodies are, therefore, deprived of nutrients that they need for optimal health.

- Calorie counting leads us to eat a far more restricted variety of foods as we avoid high calorie foods in favour of low calorie alternatives. This directly leads to Food Intolerance, as we tend to eat the same foods on a regular basis. This also leads to nutritional deficiency, as the best way to guarantee that we eat all the nutrients we need is to eat a varied diet. The foods we generally opt for on low calorie diets also tend to be those that feed Candida overgrowth – fruits, vinegary salads, crisp breads and so on.

Medication

For many people medication is the start of the vicious spiral downwards. Frequent doses of antibiotics or being on the contraceptive pill can create the right environment for Candida to proliferate. Candida causes cravings directly. Medication can also weaken the natural immune system giving rise to further Candida overgrowth, Food Intolerance or Hypoglycaemia. There is a bit of chicken and egg going on here as people generally take antibiotics because they have an infection, which can be indicative of a weakened immune system, but then the medication may weaken the immune system further.

The flow diagram just needs one route in and then the problems of cravings, weakened immune system, high consumption of carbohydrates, Candida, Food Intolerance and Hypoglycaemia all feed off each other in an explosive way. The route in is often calorie counting or medication but it can be stress…

Stress

Stress is the third major causal factor that can start off all of our problems with food and cravings. Stress has a lot to do with the way we eat in the modern world. Our busy lives lead us to eat on the run and grab convenience and fast foods rather than taking the time to prepare fresh vegetable dishes and cook some fish or meat. When we do eat protein it is often low fat cheese in a sandwich, or burger meat in a bun, or fish in breadcrumbs – we so rarely eat whole foods, simply cooked with no additives or other extras.

Stress also directly affects our blood glucose level as it has been shown that the fright, flight, fight mechanism, which helped cave people get out of dangerous situations, is still present in us today. Our adrenalin is raised not by charging animals or angry tribes, but by traffic queues and rows with our partners or children. Any adrenalin rush has been shown to impact our blood glucose level – even caffeine, which has no calories or carbohydrates, has been shown to impact our blood glucose level as it acts as a stimulant.

Hence the message here is that we are upsetting our blood glucose level throughout the day – not just with the food and drink that we consume but with caffeine and our stress levels and the way our adrenal glands still work in modern life.

Stress can also lead us to take medication, which can weaken our immune system and then set us off into the vicious circle of causes, conditions, cravings and overeating.

Stress often leads to a high consumption of carbohydrates as we turn to food for comfort. There is a medical logic for this as carbohydrates tend to be high in a substance called serotonin, which has been shown to have a strong impact on our moods. (Serotonin is the substance upon which anti-depressants act). Hence we are trying to help our bodies when we reach for carbohydrates in times of stress. The trouble is that refined carbohydrates upset our blood glucose balance and general health even further and we then end up in the vicious spiral downwards.

High consumption of carbohydrates

Still in the 'causes' section, we have a high consumption of carbohydrates as something that leads to food cravings in a number of ways. A high consumption of carbohydrates leads to:
- Candida, as it feeds the yeast,
- Food Intolerance, as we tend to eat the same carbohydrates on a regular basis,
- Hypoglycaemia, as carbohydrates directly and immediately impact our blood glucose level and stability,
- A high production of insulin, which can lead directly to overweight as insulin is the fattening hormone.

It can also weaken our immune system if we eat carbohydrates at the expense of protein and good fats.

Weakened immune system

A weakened immune system leads to:
- Candida, as it creates the environment for the yeast to multiply,
- Food Intolerance, as our bodies are more susceptible to adverse reactions to common foods,
- Hypoglycaemia, as our general health is likely to impact our blood glucose level and stability.

A weakened immune system can also lead us to take medication for infections or other health problems and this can then keep the vicious circle going.

A limited variety of foods

This directly fuels Food Intolerance and it can further weaken the immune system if the limited foods eaten do not provide the vitamins and minerals that the body needs. It is often the result of calorie counting in the first place as we tend to stick to a limited variety of low calorie foods when we count calories.

Piecing the Jigsaw together

With the flow diagram, therefore, we can see how completely interrelated a number of factors are and how all of them lead to food cravings and overeating and hence overweight. Those that stimulate insulin production, such as stress or a high consumption of carbohydrates, can lead directly to overweight as insulin facilitates the storage of fat.

If you have ever calorie counted, ever been under stress, ever taken antibiotics or hormones such as the pill... If you have sacrificed eating protein and fat in favour of carbohydrates... If you have eaten a lot of low fat, low calorie, high carbohydrate foods... If you have eaten the same foods on a regular basis... If you have a weakened immune system... If you have ever eaten a less than perfect diet... You can easily have created the environment for one, or all, of Candida, Food Intolerance and Hypoglycaemia. Any one of these will lead to addict-like food cravings, further food problems and a vicious circle of problems that make you overweight and keep you overweight.

This model explains why the more we count calories the fatter we get as we make ourselves susceptible to a multitude of problems that cause food cravings. It explains why twentieth and twenty-first century drugs and stress have led to the current epidemic of obesity. It explains why your cravings are so powerful that your desire to be slim alone cannot overcome them. It explains why you overeat when all you want is to be slim.

The good news is that the jigsaw can be used in our favour just as easily as it has worked against us in the past. Knowing what is happening, knowing why we have the cravings and knowing what causes what, we can use this knowledge to break the cycle and break free from overeating.

KEY POINTS FROM CHAPTER 12

- All the things that you may have read about do fit together in a jigsaw and they do make sense.
- There are many physical reasons why you overeat and they are all very closely connected. Calorie counting is at the heart of everything. This leads directly and indirectly to cravings and overeating.
- Other key causes are medication, stress, a high consumption of carbohydrates, a weakened immune system and eating a limited variety of foods. All of these are interlinked and have different causes and effects between them.
- All of these can lead directly and indirectly to the three conditions that cause insatiable food cravings – Candida, Food Intolerance and Hypoglycaemia.
- The outcome of all of this is cravings, overeating, excess insulin production and overweight.
- What is more, given that the causes and conditions are so interlinked, they form a vicious circle such that the worse they become the more you crave food and overeat and this worsens the conditions and the cravings further. The vicious circle is explained in more detail in Chapter 20.

PART 4

EATING & NUTRITION

PART 4

EATING & NUTRITION

Introduction

If you are reading this book I bet that you have tried all the diets around. The Atkins, Scarsdale, The Zone, Liquid meal replacements, Cabbage soup and so on. I bet you know the calorie content of almost every food and drink imaginable. I bet, over the years, you have lost and gained hundreds of pounds. We are bombarded with conflicting and confusing information – do eat potatoes, don't eat potatoes, eat carbohydrate not fat, eat fat not carbohydrate. We don't know which way to turn, whom to believe, where to start. Let's start trying to find a way through all the confusion.

First of all, let us make a bold statement – all diets in all diet books will work. If you follow the advice given in any diet book, to the letter, you will lose weight. How can this be right? Why aren't we all slim then? There are two key reasons:

1) Four key words need to be added to the statement "*all diets in all diet books will work.*" These four key words are "**in the short term.**" They do all work **in the short term** but few work in the long term, even if you could stick to them. Any diet that restricts calories, will become less and less effective in the medium to long term as your body adjusts to compensate for the calorie deficit. In the long run, almost everyone finds that they put on weight eating the same number of calories that used to make them lose weight.

2) The second key reason is that we can't stick to the diets. Liquid meal replacements, the egg and grapefruit diet (or one of its hundreds of variations) and the cabbage soup diet are not sustainable in the long term – they are not life-long ways of eating. They will help you lose weight in the short term but they will do nothing to re-educate your eating habits and they will do nothing to change the key reason why you overeat – cravings. In fact many of them will make cravings worse. The top three ingredients in Slim-Fast are water, skimmed milk powder and sucrose i.e. sugar. The sugar will ensure that your blood glucose is on a roller coaster all day long leading to strong

cravings for refined carbohydrates to elevate your blood glucose level back to normal. You may also have Food Intolerance induced cravings to either milk or sugar. Fad diets also weaken your immune system opening the door to Candida, Food Intolerance and Hypoglycaemia, which will stimulate cravings even further.

Other diets do claim to be life-long healthy eating regimes, which will help you lose weight and stay at that weight for ever, but they just don't seem practical for the majority of us and they deny us the opportunity to enjoy our food, which should be a huge pleasure in life. We cannot refute that to follow the diet of cave people (*"Neanderthin"*, for example), is something that we could do for life (cave people did it after all). However, cave people lived about a third of the average lifespan currently enjoyed in the western world and they didn't have the temptations of the taste buds that we have today. Why would you want to live like a cave person when you can have so many wonderful foods, even salads and fruits, which cave people would have longed for but could not obtain?

We can't stick to the diets because they do little to reduce our cravings and because many of them are just not workable. How can we have prawns sautéed in garlic butter for lunch, on our low carbohydrate diet, when we work in an office? Why would we have half an apple and a spoonful of cottage cheese for a mid afternoon snack when we are racing to pick the kids up from school – we would eat the whole apple and not be able to carry the cottage cheese.

We can't make them work in the long run because they are too restrictive and/or because they don't work in the long run. This leads us to a really important discovery. When you look at why diets fail, you can logically come up with an eating plan that will work.

What are the five key characteristics of a workable diet?

To be successful, that means to enable people to lose weight and to keep it off in the long term, a diet must have the following characteristics:

1) It must work and not just in the short term. It must work in the long term i.e. it must help you reach your natural weight and stay there.

2) It must be practical – a real diet for the real world. No working out grams of protein or counting calories or carbohydrates – some simple rules that you can follow at home, on holiday, at work or at play as part of your busy lifestyle.

3) It must be a long term way of eating, something you can stick to and not something you go on and then go off, leading to life-long weight fluctuations.

4) It must be healthy and deliver the nutrients you need for healthy living.

5) It must be enjoyable and not take away eating as a pleasure in life.

If we look at diets that you may have tried so far they all fall down in one or more areas. There is a summary table below. (Please note this is my own interpretation from experience and research – you may have found the cabbage soup diet most enjoyable, for example, so you can add your own ticks and crosses). The chances are, if you have found one of these to work for you in the long term you won't be reading this book anyway. Many men, for example, have found the low carbohydrate diet to be great for them. They seem to miss fruit and grains less than women. Some business people find the low carbohydrate diet somewhat practical, if they travel and eat out a lot on business, as they can have cooked breakfasts, steak and salad for lunch and lots more meat and fish for dinner. It is less practical for people working in an office or without time to cook and a lot of people, women in particular, miss the foods that are denied on low carbohydrate diets.

	Fad diet	Low carbohydrate diet	Low calorie diet	This eating plan
It works (in the long term)	✗	✓ (if you can stick to them)	✗	✓
It is practical	✗	✗	✓	✓
It is long term	✗	✓ (if…)	✗/✓	✓
It is healthy	✗	✗/✓	✗	✓
It is enjoyable	✗	✗	✗/✓	✓

Fad Diets

As you can see with fad diets they have nothing to recommend them – they work in the short term but may well contribute to weight gain in the long term as you slow down your metabolism, lose lean muscle and do other long term damage. They are rarely practical and require you to eat alone, avoid all social events and put your life on hold for the duration of the diet. They cannot be sustained in the long term. They are not healthy, as they invariably tell you to eat one food, or very few foods, to the exclusion of all others, and they are rarely enjoyable.

Low Carbohydrate Diets

Onto low carbohydrate diets, like the Atkins Diet and I'm sorry but I include the Zone in these. (The Zone is actually low carbohydrate and low calorie). With the Zone, for my frame, I am 'allowed' approximately 65g of protein and 83g of carbohydrate. This is below the minimum amounts recommended for adults in the book so, even if I take the minimum recommended for an adult of 75g of protein and 96g of carbohydrate, I can only eat approximately 10 protein blocks and 10 carbohydrate blocks throughout the day. This would equate to barely over 1000 calories a day (Indeed "*A Week in the Zone*" does say that the total calorie content for a day in the Zone is about 1200 calories).

The 10 carbohydrate blocks that I would be 'allowed', therefore, would be any of the following:
- one 4oz bowl of porridge oats made with 2 cups of milk **or**
- 5 pieces of fruit **or**
- 2.5 pita breads **or**
- 2 cups brown rice **or**
- 10 rice cakes.

If you mix carbohydrates, you could have one large salad, one large vegetable portion and probably a couple of pieces of fruit throughout the day with no other grains, milk, yoghurt or other carbohydrates. This seems to me to be a low carbohydrate and a low calorie diet in disguise. It is certainly not enough for an adult to feel nourished and satisfied.

However, **if you can stick to them**, low carbohydrate diets do work and they can work in the long term. The key is if you can stick with them of course. They also work quite well with cravings as they tend to cut out foods that cause Candida, Food Intolerance and Hypoglycaemia. However, they miss out on the practical side of things as it just isn't possible to have shrimps in butter or steak at one's office desk. The timing of meals is also too rigid for most people's lives and the idea of a snack of half an apple with a quarter cup of cottage cheese is just not practical. In terms of whether or not they are enjoyable I think this varies by person. For a carnivore that loves the idea of protein at each meal they may be enjoyable but they are very restrictive for vegetarians and they don't allow enough fruit and freedom for many to enjoy this diet.

Finally, they are very questionable on the health test as they deny people the opportunity to eat fruits and grains, which give us so many vitamins and minerals. Very low carbohydrate diets have been linked to heart disease, kidney damage, osteoporosis, halitosis (bad breath), cataracts, muscle weakness, asthma and constipation. The mere fact that they restrict a natural food like fruit, which is so delicious and has so many nutrients, is enough for me to steer well clear of them. The bottom line is that you don't need to go this far to lose weight and stay slim for ever. You can eat steak and salad, as these diets encourage, but you can also eat brown pasta & stir-fry, fruit and much more varied foods and still lose weight.

Low Calorie Diets

Low calorie diets ironically score quite well against most criteria, except that they don't work in the long run. They are practical – mostly people eat 'normal' foods but just less of them. People can eat cereal for breakfast, fruit for snacks, calorie counted sandwiches for lunch, calorie counted ready cooked meals for dinner and perhaps a calorie counted 'treat' somewhere during the day. The big problem is that people can't stick to them, as they get so hungry. Also, they do lots to stimulate, rather than eliminate, cravings (remember how calorie counting leads to more carbohydrates being consumed, a narrower variety of foods, a weakened immune system and all of these can contribute to Candida, Food Intolerance and Hypoglycaemia). Calorie controlled diets can be moderately healthy, depending on the foods chosen, but they fall down on being healthy overall as, by definition, they require you to consume less food than you actually need. They also score a mixed rating for how enjoyable they are, as they do allow you to eat what you want, which is a plus, but they restrict quantities so much that this can't be enjoyable overall.

This Eating Plan

The eating plan in this book meets all the characteristics of a successful diet:
- Number one, it works. This is probably the most important issue to the person who longs to be slim.
- It is practical – no half apples, no rigid meal times, no complex recipes, no prescribed meals to eat and nothing to count. Just some simple dos and don'ts by which you can manage your own eating to fit in with your own lifestyle.
- It is an eating plan that you can follow for life to help you reach and stay at your natural weight.
- It is healthy and nutritional – it gives you the vitamins and minerals you need for optimal health. It also advises that you avoid a particular food group that does little, if anything, for your health and nutrition.

- It is enjoyable. It frees you from cravings and lets you eat when you are hungry and when your body needs food. It allows as wide a variety of food as possible and allows 'treats' as often as your body can cope with them, once you have reached your natural weight.

There are three phases of the eating plan:
Phase 1   –   The 5 day kick-start eating plan,
Phase 2   –   The weight loss eating plan,
Phase 3   –   The life-long eating plan.
Each of the phases has three key objectives:

The 5 day kick-start eating plan is designed to do the following:

- To 'kick-start' your new way of eating with a programme that is short enough to stick to but long enough to have a significant impact on Candida, Food Intolerance and Hypoglycaemia.
- To achieve the maximum impact on food cravings (by having the maximum impact on Candida, Food Intolerance and Hypoglycaemia) when motivation and will power are highest at the start of the eating plan.
- To achieve significant weight loss.

The weight loss eating plan is designed to do the following:

- To continue to win the war against Candida, Food Intolerance and Hypoglycaemia (and thereby to have continued impact on food cravings).
- To continue the great start made in the 'kick-start' phase but with a more varied eating plan that is easier to stick to and more enjoyable.
- To change your eating habits for ever. To put you off one particular food group long term and to re-educate your palate that there is a wonderful variety of food out there which is filling, good for you and very tasty.

The life-long eating plan is designed to do the following:

- To put you back in control of your eating by giving you long term control over food cravings.
- To enable you to eat, without cravings, for life.
- To enable you to eat whatever you want **almost** whenever you want but with you managing the outcome.

You really will be able to eat whatever you want **almost** whenever you want but you will need to watch out for the warning signs, or your problems could return. You may also make the choice that you want to stay eating healthily for the rest of your life and you may, therefore, reject some of the food choices that you make currently. The key thing is that you will be free from cravings so you will not have the addict-like desire for particular foods that you have now. So you really will be able to 'take it or leave it', even with the food that you most crave right now.

13

PHASE 1

The 5 day kick-start eating plan

Introduction

I almost called this chapter the 'perfect eating plan' but this would have been misleading as there is no such thing. Every individual is different and some foods work well for some people and not for others. There is, however, a 'core' eating plan which is pretty close to being perfect for the treatment of any, or all, of Candida, Food Intolerance and Hypoglycaemia.

As I expect you're dying to know what you can eat, for how long, when, how much and why, I'll go straight into a summary of the Phase 1 eating plan.

WHAT can you eat & drink/not eat or drink in Phase 1 (in brief)?

You can eat the following: meat, fish, quorn, any salads, any vegetables (except potatoes or mushrooms) and some brown rice. You can cook in olive oil or butter or use either of these as a salad or vegetable dressing. You can also eat tofu, eggs and Natural Live Yoghurt (NLY) if you are tolerant to soy, eggs and dairy products.

You can drink still or sparkling water, herbal teas, decaffeinated tea and coffee.

You must not eat anything that is not on the list above. No fruit, no wheat or grains other than brown rice, no white rice, no sugar, no cakes, no biscuits, no confectionery, no cheese, no pickled or processed foods.

You must not drink alcohol, fruit juices, soft drinks, low calorie soft drinks, caffeinated products or milk.

HOW long is Phase 1 (in brief)?

Just five days. This is all the time you need to spend on Phase 1 for it to have a dramatic impact on your health and food cravings.

WHEN do you eat (in brief)?

Whenever you want. All the foods allowed in Phase 1 can be eaten whenever you want.

HOW much do you eat (in brief)?

As much as you want of everything on the 'allowed' list, except brown rice which should be limited to 2oz (dry weight before cooking) per day for people who eat meat or fish. Because Phase 1 is so tough for vegetarians (see Chapter 25) they should eat more brown rice (up to 6oz dry weight before cooking per day) to ensure that they don't go hungry.

WHY do you do this (in brief)?

You are following an eating plan that is just about perfect for Candida, Food Intolerance and Hypoglycaemia. You will have a significant impact on all three of these conditions in a very short period of time. Your weight loss during this short phase will also be dramatic and this will encourage you to move into Phase 2 totally committed to keeping control over your eating.

HOW will you feel (in brief)?

You may feel fine. You may quite quickly feel better than you have done for years, as the foods that are causing you problems are not put into your body. However, you do need to be aware that you may have some quite strong withdrawal symptoms and if Candida is a big problem for you, you really can feel quite unwell during Phase 1. There is more on this throughout the book. The bottom line is that the worse you feel during Phase 1, the more of the conditions of Candida, Food Intolerance and Hypoglycaemia you are likely to have had.

You probably want to know more about – what, how long for, when, how much, why, how will you feel – so let's go into these in much more detail...

WHAT can you eat & drink/not eat or drink?

The kick-start eating plan goes back to basics and assumes that you have any one, or all, of Candida, Food Intolerance and Hypoglycaemia. It cuts back to the core foods and drinks that would be allowed on all of these eating plans. It should come as no surprise that this is very similar to the diet that we would have eaten naturally, hundreds or thousands of years ago, before Candida, before Food Intolerance and before Hypoglycaemia.

The table below shows the foods that are allowed in eating plans to treat each of Candida, Food Intolerance and Hypoglycaemia. The foods and drinks that are allowed in all of the eating plans are highlighted in bold as these are the ones you can have during Phase 1.

	ALLOWED	MAYBE	NOT ALLOWED
Candida	**Any meat** **Any fish** Tofu/**Quorn** Eggs **Vegetables/salads** (Except mushrooms, potatoes) NLY **Brown rice**	Dairy products Fruit Whole-meal grains Pulses/beans all in moderation	All refined carbohydrates Yeasty foods Vinegary foods
Food Intolerance	**Any meat** **Any fish** **Quorn** **Vegetables/salads** Pulses/beans **Brown rice** Fruit Oats	* The foods in the final column are the common Food Intolerances. They may be fine for you	All refined carbohydrates Dairy Products Wheat Corn * Eggs Soy * (Tofu) Peanuts * Sugar Any food, which you consume on a regular basis
Hypoglycaemia	**Any meat** **Any fish** Tofu/**Quorn** Eggs **Vegetables/salads** Pulses/beans **Brown rice** NLY Dairy Products	Fruit Whole-meal grains Both in moderation – tune in to how sensitive your own body is to carbohydrates	All refined carbohydrates

NLY – Natural Live Yoghurt

There is, therefore, a lot of common ground on the YES and NO lists. The three foods to watch out for are tofu (soy product), eggs and Natural Live Yoghurt. If you suspect that you have Food Intolerance to any of these, you must leave them out too.

The five day eating plan should, therefore, contain the following foods:

Meat:
As much as you want of pure, unprocessed, fresh meat, no smoked or cured meat. This can include pork, bacon, fresh ham (i.e. with no preservatives or other added ingredients), beef, veal, rabbit, chicken, turkey, pheasant, quail, goose, guinea fowl, duck, lamb, venison. Please check all ingredients, as packaged and tinned meats invariably have sugars, preservatives and all sorts of things in them.

Fish:
As much as you want of pure, unprocessed, fresh fish, no smoked or cured fish. This can include white fish like plaice, haddock, turbot, and halibut and so on. It can include oily fish like mackerel, pilchards, tuna, and salmon and so on. It can include shellfish and seafood like prawns, lobster (provided of course that you don't have a food **allergy** to any fish or seafood).

You can eat tinned fish that has no added ingredients other than oil or salt. You can cook fish in olive oil or butter or steam, bake or grill it.

Eggs:
As many eggs as you want **if you are not intolerant to them**. They can be chicken, duck or any other eggs you can get hold of. Don't worry about consuming too many eggs during Phase 1 if you worry about cholesterol for example. Remember Chapter 5 on fat and what is really bad for your cholesterol – hydrogenated or transunsaturated fats – and we don't have any of these in Phase 1 (or Phase 2 for that matter).

Tofu/Quorn:
Vegetarian protein alternatives are fine if they do not contain added ingredients and if you are tolerant to soy products, of which tofu is one.

Salads & Vegetables:
- Salad ingredients – alfalfa, beetroot, celery, cress, cucumber, endive, all types of lettuce, radish, spring onions and a couple of fruits – olives and tomatoes.
- Any root vegetables – carrot, parsnip, turnip, swede.

- Other vegetables – aubergine/eggplant, asparagus, bamboo shoots, broccoli, Brussels sprouts, cabbage, cauliflower, celeriac, chillies, courgettes/zucchini, garlic, green/French beans, leek, mange tout, marrow, okra, onions, peas, peppers (any colour), pumpkin, salsify, shallots, spinach, squashes, water chestnuts.
- Any herbs, spices or seasoning – basil, coriander, chives, cumin, dill, fennel, mint, oregano, paprika, parsley, pepper, rosemary, sage, salt, thyme.

The key vegetables that are not on the above list are mushrooms and potatoes. Mushrooms feed Candida so should be avoided in Phase 1. Potatoes are too high in carbohydrate for Phase 1 as we are trying to stabilise your blood glucose level.

Be as adventurous as you can with salads and vegetables during Phase 1 (and Phase 2). You can make home-made coleslaw with cabbage (red and white), carrots, onions, celery and whatever else you fancy and you can use olive oil and/or beaten eggs as a dressing. (The eggs will make the dressing more like mayonnaise). There are some fabulous aubergine/eggplant recipes at the back of this book. (Leave out the cheese in these recipes for Phase 1). You can stir-fry vegetables in olive oil and have a Chinese stir-fry with your brown rice or have a tomato/onion/garlic based sauce for your rice or meat dishes. Make Phase 1 as varied and enjoyable as you possibly can.

Natural Live Yoghurt (NLY):
Unless you are intolerant to dairy products you can have NLY in Phase 1. Remember from Chapter 9 the great benefit you can get from NLY in the war on Candida. Try a goat's or sheep's version of live yoghurt, if you are sensitive to milk, as the health benefits of live yoghurt for Candida and the digestive tract are so significant.

Brown rice:
You can have up to 2oz (dry weight – before cooking) of brown rice per day – no rice cakes instead as they are full of air and are, in effect, refined. If you are vegetarian or vegan you can have up to 6oz (dry weight before cooking) of brown rice per day to make sure you get enough to eat.

Do not eat anything that is not on the above list during Phase 1 – no fruit, no other grains, no milk, cheese or other dairy products. You may drink as much bottled or filtered water and herbal teas as you like during Phase 1, but no alcohol, caffeine or canned drinks (even low calorie drinks) or fruit juices.

Below are some meal options for Phase 1. There are some more meal options in Chapter 14 where I specify which of them are suitable for people suffering from Candida, Food Intolerance and Hypoglycaemia and which are suitable for Phase 1. There are recipes in Part 10 for the following meal options marked with an (R):

Breakfasts:
- Bacon & eggs,
- Scrambled eggs (no milk) (R) – cooked in butter and flavoured with salt and pepper as desired,
- Plain or ham Omelette (no milk) (R) – cooked in butter and flavoured with salt and pepper as desired,
- NLY (you can have a few sunflower, or other, seeds mixed in),
- Kedgeree (fish and brown rice).

Main meals (lunch/dinner):
- Asparagus in butter,
- Char-grilled Vegetables with olive oil dressing (R),
- Vegetable kebabs,
- A selection of soups (R),
- Salade niçoise (R),
- Salmon niçoise (R),
- Any amount of meat & salad/vegetables,
- Any amount of fish or seafood & salad/vegetables,
- Omelette & salad (R),
- Egg and/or cold meat salad,
- Meat & stir-fry vegetables,
- Quorn & vegetables in home-made tomato sauce (R for the tomato sauce),
- Roast leg of lamb with rosemary & vegetables (R),
- Roast chicken with garlic or lemon (R),
- Stuffed tomatoes (R),
- Stuffed peppers (R),
- Brown rice with stir-fry vegetables (R for the stir-fry),
- Tofu & stir-fry vegetables (R for the stir-fry),
- Butternut squash curry & brown rice (R),
- Aubergine/eggplant boats (see the recipe in Part 10 and leave out the cheese).

HOW long is Phase 1?

Phase 1 lasts for just five days. Five short days to kick-start your eating habits and the fight against food cravings.

Why five days? This very strict part of the eating plan needs to be short enough for you to stick to it but long enough to have an effect. In just twenty-four to forty-eight hours you can make dramatic changes to your blood glucose stability. In three to four days, any substance to which you have been intolerant will have passed through your system and you will start to feel free from the cravings that this food has generated. Candida is the one condition that isn't 'fixed' in five days, but you can still make a big difference with it in five days. You will continue to fight Candida during the second phase of the eating plan, but the very strict phase should be kept as short as possible so that you can stick to it.

You can continue this eating plan beyond five days if you are suffering from all three conditions, have much weight to lose and can identify with the majority of the symptoms in the chapters on Candida, Food Intolerance and Hypoglycaemia. However, as the weight loss plan in the next chapter is merely an extension of this eating plan (with more foods added for variety and nutrients) you may also be fine moving to the next phase.

WHEN do you eat?

You can eat whenever you want. All the foods allowed in Phase 1 can be eaten whenever you want. It is best to get into the habit of eating three main meals a day with in between meal snacks only if you are genuinely hungry. However, the most important thing with Phase 1 is to complete it, so eat whenever you want to make sure you are not hungry and can stick to the eating plan for the full five days.

HOW much do you eat?

As much as you want of everything on the 'allowed' list except brown rice, which should be limited to 2oz (dry weight before cooking) per day for people who eat meat or fish. Because Phase 1 is so tough for vegetarians (see Chapter 25) they should eat more brown rice (up to 6oz dry weight before cooking per day) to ensure that they don't go hungry.

You really can have a large plate of bacon and eggs for breakfast (just make sure the bacon has no added ingredients) and you can have as much meat, fish, salad and vegetables as you can eat for main meals.

If you need to snack between your three main meals then you can have cold meats, hard-boiled eggs, celery sticks, raw carrots, Natural Live Yoghurt or a tin of tuna – whatever it takes to keep hunger at bay. **WHY do you do this?**

Phase 1 is designed to achieve the following:
- To 'kick-start' your new way of eating with a programme that is short enough to stick to but long enough to have a significant impact on Candida, Food Intolerance and Hypoglycaemia.
- To achieve the maximum impact on food cravings (by having the maximum impact on Candida, Food Intolerance and Hypoglycaemia) when motivation and will power are highest at the start of the eating plan.
- To achieve significant weight loss.

The logic for the five day eating plan is as follows – we simply take the eating plans recommended for each of the conditions of Candida, Food Intolerance and Hypoglycaemia and we identify the definite yes's (what is allowed), definite no's (what is not allowed) and the maybe's. We can see that there is a lot of common ground for each of the eating plans. Please note that with Food Intolerance, any food can cause a problem for an individual but the foods listed are generally the foods that rarely cause problems for the majority of people. If any of the foods listed in the YES category do cause you problems (e.g. tomatoes under salads) then don't eat this food. Remember the best way to tell if a food is a problem for you is to be honest about whether you crave it or not. Sadly the foods we most want are the foods we must avoid – just in the short term until they become OK to consume again.

The benefits of the five day eating plan are:
- It is strict when your willpower is highest – at the start of the eating plan.
- It should be completely different to anything that you have tried before, which will jolt your body into action.
- You will see dramatic weight loss in just five days, despite the fact that you will not be counting calories at all.
- You will see your cravings subside each day – by day four or five they should be much more tolerable.
- You will rid your body of all the foods, to which you are intolerant, that have been causing your ill health.
- You will get your blood glucose back under control straight away.
- You will make a huge start in the fight against Candida – the yeast will have had a major attack in just a few days and will have started

118

to die off. The ground work will have been done for getting your gut flora back in balance.

HOW will you feel?

The idea behind this eating plan is that you will cut out, for just five days, all foods that could contribute to Candida, Food Intolerance and Hypoglycaemia.

- If Candida has been your problem you will start to feel some quite dramatic and unpleasant symptoms as the Candida is killed off in your body. This reaction has been called 'Herxheimer's' reaction or 'Candida-die-off'.
- If you have suffered any Food Intolerance then you will notice immense withdrawal symptoms and quite unbelievable cravings for the first three to four days as the food is missed by your body. Once the offending substances have passed through your body, you will start to experience a physical well-being and mental clarity that you have possibly not felt in years.
- If Hypoglycaemia has been your problem then, within just twenty-four to forty-eight hours, your blood glucose level will stabilise and again you will experience a physical well-being and mental clarity that you have possibly not felt in years.

The next thing I can guarantee is that you will crave food! In this first five days, the Candida will be screaming at you to feed it. Every food to which you are intolerant will be calling out to you *'eat me'* and your hypoglycaemic body will be asking for a sugar high. The other thing I can guarantee is that your mind will start playing games with you. On the first day of Phase 1, the cravings will come out in force and your mind will start making unhelpful suggestions. The key one it will make is *"go on – have the food you want today. You can start this diet thing tomorrow."* Sounds familiar? The trouble is – how is it going to be any easier tomorrow? The same excuse can be made tomorrow and the day after and the day after that and this is why you are still overeating and overweight when you have wanted to be slim for years. You have to start now. Don't waste another day of your life. A key thing to remember is that Candida, Food Intolerance and Hypoglycaemia don't get better. They get worse by the day. So, if you do give in today and vow to start tomorrow, it will be even more difficult tomorrow. If you think today is tough, tackle it now before it gets any tougher.

This five day eating plan will kick-start your life-long change in eating habits. It will be cleansing and cathartic but it will also require all the willpower you have left to get to the end of the five days. You will essentially be going 'cold turkey' like a drug addict – not by giving up food but by giving up the foods to which you have been addicted. Pick the time you do this carefully, get friends and family to support if necessary. You may feel so unwell with the withdrawal symptoms and Candida-die-off that you may even be off work with 'sickness'. The die-off may lead to a worsening of your previous symptoms of Candida, particularly the foggy brain feeling, lack of concentration and muscle weakness. Hence don't start in the week when you have a key meeting or event to attend. A good option, if you can't afford to take time off, is to start the five day kick-start eating plan on a Thursday and struggle through until the weekend, rest and recover over Saturday and Sunday and then by Monday you should be starting to feel quite a bit better.

The length of the die-off reaction depends on the severity of the original yeast infection, upon your current diet and on how well your body is able to detoxify. Usually any reaction begins within a few hours of starting an anti-Candida diet and it may last for a couple of weeks in the worst cases but each case is unique. It is really important to stick to the anti-Candida diet, if you do get these symptoms, as this is proof that you have been suffering from an extreme Candida overgrowth. During the die-off you can help the detoxification process by drinking lots of water, eating lots of vegetables and salads (high fibre) and taking a vitamin & mineral supplement. Many people will get through the five days feeling fine but you should be warned of the worst extreme in case it happens to you and you think you are going down with the flu.

Just a final thought – you may benefit from speeding up the passage of foods to which you may be intolerant through your system during this five day period. Without being too graphic, if there is a food that always makes you go to the loo then this may be a good idea for the last day before you start the programme! This may be curry. I know someone for whom this is aubergine/eggplant. The faster we can work those offending foods through your system, the better.

Top tips for inspiration

This is just five short days that could change your life for ever.

You will make a dramatic difference to all the conditions of Candida, Food Intolerance and Hypoglycaemia during even this brief time.

You will balance your blood glucose level and have a huge impact on Hypoglycaemia.

You will rid your body of all the foods to which you have become intolerant.

You will make a great start in the attack on Candida to get this hideous parasite back under control in your body.

If you feel dreadful at all during the five days, this is a fantastic sign that you have had quite significant problems with the three conditions and you are making real progress.

If you feel OK, then be thankful that you have caught these conditions before they have become really bad.

No matter how you feel during the five days, you will have a clear head and mental clarity at the end of the five days that you may not have had for years.

You have to do this some time so you may as well do it now. The longer you leave it, the worse the conditions will become and the nastier the five day onslaught will be when you finally do get round to it.

KEY POINTS FROM CHAPTER 13

- **Do eat** meat, fish, eggs, (tofu – if you are tolerant to soy products), quorn, Natural Live Yoghurt, any salads, any vegetables (except potatoes or mushrooms), some brown rice, herbs & spices, olive oil and butter.
- **Do drink** still or sparkling water, herbal teas, decaffeinated tea or coffee.
- **Don't eat** anything that is not on the list above. No fruit, no wheat or grains other than brown rice, no white rice, no sugar, no cakes, no biscuits, no confectionery, no cheese, no pickled or processed foods.
- **Don't drink** alcohol, fruit juices, soft drinks, low calorie soft drinks, caffeinated products or milk.
- Follow all of the above for just five days.
- Eat whenever you want – three meals a day is ideal but the key thing is not to get hungry.
- Eat as much as you want of everything on the 'allowed' list except brown rice, which is restricted.
- Do this because you are following just about the perfect eating plan for all three of Candida, Food Intolerance and Hypoglycaemia.
- During the five days you may feel great, you may feel fine, you may feel pretty rough. The key thing is that by the end of the five days you should be starting to feel better than you have for years.

14

PHASE 2

The weight loss eating plan

Introduction

The key thing about Phase 2 is that it has to be workable. I have read all the diet books, just like you have, that say you must eat 2oz of home-made muesli and half a glass of skimmed milk at breakfast with chopped dried fruit pieces; a quarter cup of cottage cheese and half an apple for a mid morning snack; pan seared chicken with pasta salad and 2 tablespoons of home-made dressing and sautéed red snapper on black bean relish for dinner, with the recipe page references everywhere. Where is the person who can make this work for them? Everyone I know is struggling with a job, a family, studying, or all three. I don't know anyone who even has the time to shop this prescriptively, let alone do all the preparation and then eat it at the right time on the right day.

We have to be pragmatic and recognise that we all lead incredibly busy lives and we just don't have the time, or the energy, to be this black and white about our eating. What we need then are some general guidelines, which should tell us what to eat and what not to eat, but as little as possible about when and how and in what quantities.

WHAT can you eat & drink/not eat or drink in Phase 2 (in brief)?

You can eat anything on the following list below **except** anything that you have identified is a problem for you personally – we will go into this in more depth after the 'in brief' section.

You can eat:

- Fat/Protein – meat, fish, eggs, (tofu – if you are tolerant to soy products), quorn, cheese, milk, dairy products and Natural Live Yoghurt.

- Carbohydrates – any fruits, any salads, any vegetables, baked jacket potatoes, any whole-meal grains (brown rice, brown pasta, and whole-wheat bread with no refined ingredients). Any beans & pulses (chick peas, kidney beans, broad beans, lentils etc).

- Fats – olive oil, sunflower oil, other vegetable oils, butter.

- Drinks – still or sparkling water, herbal teas, decaffeinated tea & coffee and an occasional glass of red wine with meals (more on this later).

You must not eat anything that is not on the list above. No white grains (white rice, white pasta, white bread or brown bread with refined ingredients). No sugar, no cakes, no biscuits, no confectionery or processed foods.

You must not drink fruit juices, soft drinks or low calorie soft drinks. Caffeine and alcohol should ideally be avoided but we have a particular note on these below as total avoidance of caffeine and red wine could be too much for some people.

HOW long is Phase 2 (in brief)?

For as long as you want to lose weight.

WHEN do you eat (in brief)?

Whenever you want. Ideally just three meals a day but if you are genuinely hungry and need snacks in between meals then have them.

HOW much do you eat (in brief)?

As much as you want but there is one rule about mixing different types of food. This will be spelled out in detail after the 'in brief' section.

WHY do you do this (in brief)?

In brief, Phase 2 is designed to meet all the characteristics of a successful eating plan:
- Phase 2 works. You will lose weight.
- Phase 2 is practical.
- Phase 2 can be followed in the long term to help you reach and stay at your natural weight.
- Phase 2 is healthy and nutritious.
- Phase 2 is enjoyable.

HOW will you feel (in brief)?

You will feel fantastic! You will not be hungry. You will be free from cravings. You will be eating real healthy foods which will be nourishing your body and giving you energy like you've not had for years. You can eat both carbohydrate and fat/protein (just not at the same time) so you should not feel deprived. You will be able to eat out and dine in, snack and lose weight, at the same time as keeping your busy lifestyle.

As we did in the last chapter, let us go into – what, how, when and why – in much more detail. We need to really understand how we can eat so much and lose weight.

WHAT can you eat & drink/not eat or drink in Phase 2?

The Phase 2 eating plan has just three rules. Get to know them as well as your best friend as these are going to be your secret to a life-long way of eating healthily and staying at your natural weight.

Please note that these 'rules' are for Phase 2 only – ideally you will adopt them as the basis of a life-long way of eating but you can go back to eating anything in Phase 3 (yes anything!) but you will have to keep a close eye on how each food makes you feel and take control again quickly if cravings return.

RULE NUMBER 1
Don't eat refined carbohydrates.

Remember, refined carbohydrates are all carbohydrates that have been altered in some way from their natural form. Unrefined carbohydrates are all carbohydrates that are eaten as they would be found in their natural form. So, always eat the whole food, don't eat refined carbohydrates.

This means:

- don't eat sugar in any form – white or brown – or any of its derivatives e.g. sucrose, glucose syrup, corn syrup, maltose, fructose, dextrose etc. (anything with "*ose*" at the end). Please note, sugar is found in cakes, biscuits, confectionery, almost every cereal, most crisp breads, many crisps, most desserts and many types of yoghurt.

- don't eat white rice as this is refined from brown rice.

- don't eat white pasta as this is refined from whole-wheat pasta.

- don't eat white bread (also no brown bread with any refined ingredients like sugar, honey or treacle).

- don't drink fruit juice (as fruit juice is just refined fruit).

- don't eat dried fruit (as dried fruit is also refined fruit).

- don't eat chips, crisps, fries (as these are refined potatoes).

Look out for refined carbohydrates in the most unexpected places. Spend an extra hour in a supermarket one day and read every label of the products you normally purchase – you will be astonished at what contains sugar. I have seen sugar in cottage cheese, dextrose in packets of ham, treacle in whole-wheat bread, sugar and bread in crab fish sticks and you may find many more when you become vigilant. On the following page is a summary table to show where you will find refined carbohydrates:

FOOD	UNREFINED – GOOD	REFINED – BAD
GRAINS	Brown rice Whole-wheat pasta Whole-wheat flour Whole-wheat bread (without sugar, glucose syrup, treacle & other refined carbohydrates)	White rice White pasta White flour White bread or any bread with sugar or sugar substances in it.
FRUITS	Any whole fruits (eating the skins where edible)	Dried fruits e.g. dates Fruit juices
VEGETABLES	Baked potatoes with the skins on Any other vegetables	Chips, crisps, fries Vegetable juices, dried vegetables (vegetable crisps)
MEAT	Any pure meat with no food processing e.g. pork chops, steak, lamb joints, carvery meat etc. Any meat from the butchers or the fresh meat counter in the grocery store.	Processed meats e.g. burgers, sausages Tinned meats often have ingredients added - check the label. Sliced packaged meats invariably have sugar/dextrose in them.
FISH	Any fish from the fishmongers or the fresh fish counter in the grocery store. Most tinned fish is OK - tuna, salmon, sardines - check the labels.	Processed fish - fish fingers, fish in breadcrumbs (contains white bread and sugar).
SUGAR	Any sugar found naturally in whole food: fruit sugar in the whole fruit; milk sugar in milk.	Any refined sugar white or brown; maltose, dextrose, sucrose, fructose added to products; treacle; honey * etc.
DRINKS	Water, milk, herbal teas	Canned drinks, fruit juice

* NB honey is not OK – it is a refined product

RULE NUMBER 2
Don't eat anything that will perpetuate any of the three conditions that you are suffering from.

The foods that will perpetuate (keep going) any of the three conditions that you are suffering from are almost always the foods that you crave. Remember you have to stop the cravings to stop overeating. Rule Number 2 means:

- **Candida** – Don't eat yeasty, sugary, vinegary foods if Candida is a problem for you as these foods will perpetuate Candida.

- **Food Intolerance** – Don't eat foods to which you are intolerant as these foods will perpetuate Food Intolerance. These are the foods that you crave. Identify these foods with the help of Chapter 10 and avoid the offending foods for Phase 1 and 2. Food Intolerances do change over time so you should find that you can re-introduce your problem foods over time provided that you don't return to having too much of them on a regular basis.

- **Hypoglycaemia** – Don't eat foods that upset your blood glucose balance as these foods will perpetuate Hypoglycaemia. For example, you are allowed fruit in Phase 2 but if you are particularly sensitive to sweet fruits, such as tropical fruits (bananas, melons, pineapple, mango etc), then don't eat these.

RULE NUMBER 3
Don't eat fat and carbohydrate at the same meal.

Eat either a fat meal or a carbohydrate meal but don't mix the two. The exception is that salads and green vegetables have a very small carbohydrate content and can, therefore, be eaten with either fat or carbohydrate meals. Hence your meals should be fat meals (e.g. meat, fish, cheese, eggs) with salad and/or green vegetables **or** carbohydrate meals (brown rice, brown pasta, baked potato) with salad and/or green vegetables. Coloured vegetables, like carrots, aubergine/eggplant and butternut squash, as a general rule, have a higher carbohydrate content so they should be eaten sparingly with fat meals.

The other two foods to watch are milk and nuts. If you remember from Chapter 2, these are the products in the middle of the three circles diagram. Milk and nuts contain significant amounts of carbohydrate, fat and protein. Skimmed milk is a carbohydrate and a protein with very little fat but full fat milk is, as its name suggests, also a fat. Hence don't drink full fat milk in Phase 2. As skimmed milk is not really a fat you can have this with whole-meal, sugar-free, cereals as a carbohydrate meal. For the same reason, don't eat nuts in Phase 2 because they are both carbohydrate and fat.

I have been asked how soon after a fat meal you can have a carbohydrate meal, or vice versa. The general guideline is three to four hours because this is how long it normally takes for food to be digested. You should achieve this naturally by having three meals a day but, if you are eating snacks, you need to leave three to four hours between eating a fat snack and a carbohydrate meal, or vice versa.

I have seen diet books with over twenty rules which are just far too many for any of us to take on board. None of us would ever succeed with twenty New Year's resolutions and the same applies to a change in eating habits. The three rules above are all that you need to get in control and stay in control of your eating and to reach and stay at your natural weight. Stick them on your fridge, put them in your wallet, say them as you fall asleep – do whatever it takes to get them ingrained in your mind.

The basic eating plan is in the table opposite. The table automatically covers Rule 1 as there are no refined carbohydrates anywhere. The table is then designed to help you with Rule 2:

* Take care to read all labels for sugar, treacle, honey and other hidden sugars. Ideally buy whole-wheat bread or oats from a health food shop where the ingredients are simple or bake your own bread.

BASIC EATING PLAN	NOTES FOR OTHER CONDITIONS
PROTEIN – ANIMAL Any meat or fish	All fine for Candida & Hypoglycaemia. Food Intolerance – avoid any meat or fish to which you are intolerant (rare).
PROTEIN – VEGETARIAN Beans, pulses, tofu, quorn	Candida – eat beans & pulses in moderation. Food Intolerance – avoid any of these foods to which you are intolerant (tofu perhaps). Hypoglycaemia – eat beans & pulses in moderation.
DAIRY PRODUCTS Cheese, milk, eggs, NLY	Candida – eat lots of NLY and no more than 1-2 portions per day of other dairy products. Food Intolerance – avoid any of these foods to which you are intolerant All fine for Hypoglycaemia.
CARBS. – GRAINS Any whole-meal grains – brown rice, brown pasta, quinoa, brown bread *, porridge oats (* see previous page)	Candida – eat brown rice & quinoa in moderation. Food Intolerance – avoid any grains to which you are intolerant (wheat is the most likely). Hypoglycaemia – eat whole-meal carbohydrates in moderation and never too large a portion at one sitting. Get to know what works best for you.
CARBS. – FRUITS Go easy on fruits with high sugar content and eat the rest liberally. See the list on the next page	Candida – eat no more than 1-2 portions per day from the 'lower sugar' list on the next page e.g. apples. Food Intolerance – avoid any fruits to which you are intolerant (rare). Hypoglycaemia – eat fruit in moderation and never too large a portion at one sitting.
CARBS. – VEGETABLES Eat an abundance of salads and vegetables. Eat potatoes in moderation	Candida & Hypoglycaemia – eat an abundance of salads and vegetables. Eat potatoes in moderation. Food Intolerance – avoid any vegetables to which you are intolerant (corn & tomatoes perhaps).
DRINKS Water, herbal teas, the odd glass of wine, milk, coffee & tea (ideally decaf).	Candida – drink lots of water & herbal teas. Food Intolerance – avoid any drinks to which you are intolerant (milk and coffee are the most common). Hypoglycaemia – avoid caffeine.

- If you don't think Candida, Food Intolerance or Hypoglycaemia are problems for you (you were simply overeating because you were calorie counting and hungry) then go straight for the basic eating plan in the first column.

- If you have a problem with Candida (you will know this from the questionnaire in Chapter 9 and from how ill you felt during Phase 1) then follow the Candida advice in the second column. This is very similar to the basic eating plan but it also advises you to eat beans, pulses, brown rice and quinoa in moderation (no more than 1 portion a day) and to have just 1-2 small portions of dairy products and fruit per day. Candida is the toughest of the three conditions to have and, therefore, it has the most restricted eating plan to cure it. As soon as you get to the point that your Candida is feeling well under control (redo the questionnaire in Chapter 9 as a test) you can start eating more of the foods in the basic eating plan and eat dairy products, fruit and whole-meal grains more freely.

- If there is any food to which you are intolerant, then avoid this food in Phase 2. A great way to be sure of the food(s) to which you are intolerant is to try foods that you suspect are a problem for you **on their own** immediately after doing Phase 1, the kick-start eating plan. If you eat wheat on its own for example (as plain shredded wheat cereal) after avoiding it for five days you should have a pretty rapid reaction telling you whether or not it is OK for you. If you have a return of any of the symptoms that you used to suffer (bloating, upset stomach, headaches, for example) then you will know that this is one of your problem foods and you need to avoid it for the rest of Phase 2. If you suspect milk, have a glass of milk on its own and see what happens. The eating plan for Food Intolerance is quite simple – avoid any food causing you problems. After a few weeks of avoiding the food, try it on its own and if the symptoms return you are not ready to re-introduce it. If there are no symptoms then you can eat it again, but don't have too much, or have it too often, or the intolerance will return.

- If Hypoglycaemia is a problem for you (from the check list in Chapter 11) then you can eat dairy products freely but watch your consumption of grains and fruits as these may upset your blood glucose level. Try to avoid the very sweet fruits (these are listed below) as these will have the most impact on your blood glucose level.

- If you have more than one condition you will need to follow the advice for all the conditions that affect you. This will restrict the foods that you can eat, but this is only until your immune system recovers and your body can tolerate a wider variety of foods again. You are not giving up these foods for ever.

Fruits:

This list is particularly for those people with Candida and/or Hypoglycaemia:

Lower sugar	Moderate sugar	High sugar content
Apples	Kiwi	Bananas
Pears	Grapes	Melons
Peaches/nectarines		Dates (fresh not dried)
Cherries/plums		Papaya
Blueberries/blackberries		Pineapple
Raspberries/strawberries		Sharon fruit
Citrus fruits – oranges/grapefruits etc.		Mango

If there is a fruit not listed above use your common sense as to where it should go. The best fruits for you to eat are generally staple fruits in each supermarket like apples, pears and oranges. The fruits to eat only occasionally are tropical fruits which are less frequently available.

So what do you eat on a daily basis? The next table is based on the basic eating plan but there are notes to show how it can be adapted for Candida (C in the table), Food Intolerance (FI) and Hypoglycaemia (H). The following table also brings in the final rule – Rule 3 – as it shows you how to choose either a fat meal or a carbohydrate meal...

131

TIME OF DAY	FAT OPTION	CARBOHYDRATE OPTION	DRINKS
First thing		As much fruit as you like on the basic eating plan or 1 portion (C), low sugar fruits in moderation (H)	Water, herbal tea. Coffee or tea (decaffeinated to reduce blood glucose stimulus)
Breakfast	Bacon, eggs, ham, omelettes – as much meat or fish as you like with no carbohydrate	100% whole-wheat cereal e.g. shredded wheat or porridge oats with skimmed or semi milk if desired. Or, whole-wheat bread on its own or with sugar free preserves. (NB wheat is a common FI)	Try to avoid drinks during meals as this has been shown to affect digestion.
Mid morning or mid afternoon snacks (if needed)	Cheese or boiled egg on its own	Fruit Don't go over two portions of lower sugar fruits per day for (C)	Drink as much water as possible during the day. Drink tea and coffee (decaf) in moderation. No sugar of course. (NB milk is a common FI)
Lunch	Any fish, meat, eggs, cheese – as much as you want with salad and/or vegetables but no fruit or grains	Whole-meal carbohydrates & vegetables	Try to avoid drinks during meals as this has been shown to affect digestion.
Dinner	As lunch	As lunch	As lunch

Please note that you can choose whether to have a fat meal or a carb meal whenever you like – you may like every meal to be a fat meal or every meal to be a carb meal – or any combination in between. I recommend at least one fat meal and one carb meal a day for variety.

Here are a number of different possible breakfasts and main meals – either fat options or carbohydrate options. There is a code after each meal to indicate what the meal is suitable for:

C = suitable for Candida
H = suitable for Hypoglycaemia
P1 = suitable for Phase 1 as well as Phase 2
R = the recipe for this is in Part 10
V = suitable for vegetarians

It is difficult to indicate which meals are OK for sufferers of Food Intolerance as some people may be intolerant to wheat, others to milk, others to corn and so on. If you know that there is a food to which you are intolerant then obviously don't choose the meal options which contain that food.

It is also a bit difficult to indicate which meals are OK for Hypoglycaemia as some people may be able to tolerate more fruit or grains than others. Again, please adjust the meal list according to your own needs.

Breakfasts

FAT OPTIONS	CARBOHYDRATE OPTIONS
-Full English breakfast (C, H, P1, R) -Kippers/smoked haddock (H) -Scrambled eggs (C, H, P1, R, V) -Plain omelette (C, H, P1, R, V) -Ham omelette (C, H, P1, R) -NLY (C, H, P1, V) Please note cooking options for fat breakfasts include grilling, poaching, steaming, baking or frying in butter or vegetable oil.	-Fruit platters (C, H, R, V) -Fruit and very low fat natural yoghurt (C, H, V) (Please note, fruit is OK in moderation for C and H in Phase 2) -Shredded Wheat & milk (H, V) (add a sliced banana for sweetness) -Sugar free porridge with water or milk (skimmed or semi) (C in moderation, H, V) -Sugar free muesli with water or milk (skimmed or semi) (H, V) -Whole-wheat bread & sugar free preserves (H, V)

Main Meals – Starters

FAT OPTIONS	CARBOHYDRATE OPTIONS
-Salmon & cream cheese (C, H) * -Tomatoes & Mozzarella (C, H, V) -Asparagus in butter (C, H, P1, V)	-Char-grilled vegetables with balsamic (No balsamic vinegar for P1) or olive oil dressing (C, H, P1, R, V)* -Vegetable kebabs (C, H, P1, V) -Fruit salad (C, H, V) (Get used to having fruit before the main course)* -A selection of soups (C, H, P1, R, V)
* if Candida is a problem for you *Smoked* salmon is best avoided, skip the balsamic and count the fruit salad as your 1-2 portions for the day.	

Main Meals – Main Courses

FAT OPTIONS	CARBOHYDRATE OPTIONS
-Salade niçoise (C, H, P1, R) -Salmon niçoise (C, H, P1, R) -Any meat & salad/vegetables (C, H, P1) -Any fish & salad/vegetables (C, H, P1) -Omelette & salad (C, H, P1, V, R) -Cheese, ham, egg, cold meat salad (C, H) -Cheesy leeks (C, H, R, V) -Cauliflower cheese (C, H, R, V) -Meat & stir-fry vegetables (C, H, P1) -Quorn & vegetables in tomato sauce (C, H, P1, V) -Aubergine bake (C, H, R, V) -Aubergine boats (C, H, R, V) -Roast leg of lamb with rosemary & vegetables (C, H, P1, R) -Roast chicken with garlic or lemon (C, H, P1, R) -Four cheese salad (C, H, R, V)	-Brown rice with stir-fry vegetables (C, H, P1, R, V) -Quinoa with stir-fry vegetables (C, H, R, V) -Whole-wheat pasta and tomato sauce (C, H, R, V) -Whole-wheat spaghetti and tomato sauce (C, H, R, V) -Vegetarian chilli and brown rice (C, H, R, V) -Whole-wheat cous-cous and Char-grilled vegetables (C, H, R, V) -Whole-wheat cous-cous and chick peas in coriander sauce (C, H, R, V) -Butternut squash curry & brown rice (C, H, P1, R, V) -Lentil moussaka (C, H, R, V) -Brown bread salad sandwich (H, V) -Baked potato & salad or very low fat cottage cheese (C, H, V) -Roasted vegetables with pine nuts & Parmesan cheese (C, H, R, V) -Stuffed tomatoes (C, H, P1, R, V) -Stuffed peppers (C, H, P1, R, V)

Main Meals – Desserts

FAT OPTIONS	CARBOHYDRATE OPTIONS
-Strawberries & Cream (C, H, V) -Sugar free ice cream (C, H, R, V) -NLY (C, H, P1, V) -Cheese selection (C, H, V) (NB – you can have a couple of sugar free oat biscuits with cheese)	-Berry compote (C, H, R, V) -Fruit puree (R, V)

Easy Lunches for Work on the Run

FAT OPTIONS	CARBOHYDRATE OPTIONS
-Tinned tuna/salmon with salad in a lunch box (C, H, P1) -Cuts of cold meat (chicken, turkey, beef, ham – any combination with salad) (C, H, P1) -Any leftovers from dinner the night before.	-Baked potato & salad or very low fat cottage cheese (C, H, V) -Fruit salad (C, H, V) Remember to take care with high carbohydrates such as potatoes or fruit with Hypoglycaemia.

Snacks

FAT OPTIONS	CARBOHYDRATE OPTIONS
-Cheese (C, H, V) -Hard Boiled eggs (C, H, P1, V) -Natural Live Yoghurt (C, H, P1,V)	-Sugar free cereal bars – Dr Gillian McKeith's are recommended (H, V) -Fruit (C, H, V)

Just a final word on drinks in this 'what do you eat' section...

We have said that this eating plan must be workable so there are two areas where you can 'cheat' in Phase 2 to help it work for you:

1) There are some people who just cannot face the thought of starting the day without an espresso or regular coffee or a cup of tea. There are a number of points to make here:

  - Take care that it really is the coffee/tea that you are so keen to have and not a craving for milk, which could be a sign of milk Food Intolerance.
  - Try and switch to decaffeinated alternatives if at all possible.
  - If you are not craving milk, you loathe decaf. and you really want that first espresso of the day, then have it. The key thing is that you stick to this eating plan so, if a coffee or a cup of tea in the

morning would make the difference between you sticking to this eating plan or giving up, then have one.
- However, make sure you don't go over 1, maximum 2, cup(s) a day. Ideally have them before early afternoon otherwise they will disturb your sleep patterns later that night.
- Have your early morning coffee with a carbohydrate breakfast, rather than a fat breakfast, as the caffeine will elevate your blood glucose level and you don't want that insulin in your body looking for a fat breakfast to store.
- Be aware that caffeine will give you a short term high followed by an energy low so have a strategy for getting your blood glucose level back to normal without reaching for refined carbohydrates. One case study I worked with had his espresso as soon as he woke up and then had his sugar free muesli with milk after showering so that the healthy breakfast naturally raised his blood glucose level back to normal after the caffeine high.

2) The other thing that some people just can't do without is a glass of wine with dinner. There are similar points to make here too:
- Take care that you are not craving the specific ingredients in wine and feeding Candida and/or a specific Food Intolerance. If Candida is a problem for you then you must avoid wine until this condition is back under control.
- Try and drink dry and organic wines as much as possible to limit the sweetness and additives that you consume.
- If this will make the difference with you sticking to the eating plan then have an occasional glass of wine, ideally red, with your main meal of the day.

It is obviously better in Phase 2 not to drink caffeine or wine but the key thing is to stick to the eating plan.

HOW long is Phase 2?

You should follow Phase 2 for as long as you want to lose weight. If you have a stone (14lb) or less to lose then you could easily lose 3-5lb in Phase 1 and you may only need to follow Phase 2 for a couple more weeks. If you have a great deal of weight to lose then you know you can be free from hunger and food cravings throughout Phase 2 and you will lose weight whilst eating really healthy, natural foods which will be most welcome to your body.

We should note here that if you are doing well on Phase 2 and you have a special event coming up you may like to dip into Phase 3 for a while and just maintain your weight during this occasion. The beauty of this eating plan is that it is so flexible you can eat in hotels and away on holiday or at weddings but you may want a bit more freedom for a particular occasion before reaching your natural weight. If this is the case, then read the guidelines for Phase 3 and take this ammunition along to your special occasion. The guidelines say 1) don't cheat too much 2) don't cheat too often and 3) be alert and stay in control. If you want to eat what you like at a wedding or party, therefore, follow the Phase 2 rules right up to the minute the event starts, then eat a bit of what you fancy but don't stuff yourself until you feel awful (i.e. don't cheat too much). Then don't look for every opportunity during the occasion to keep cheating. This means have the nice dinner but don't eat everything at the optional, evening buffet (i.e. don't cheat too often). Finally, be alert and stay in control.

The experience will be very interesting for you to learn from – how did you feel after eating refined carbohydrates? Was the way you felt worth the lapse? Treat everything as a learning experience as you get to know your body in a new, healthy way. (Please note the old 'good day/bad day you' might have starved up until the big event and then eaten everything in sight on the day and struggled to fight the bloating and tight clothes that followed. Because you no longer have 'good' days and 'bad' days, you know that a big wedding meal does not turn that day into a 'bad' day).

The other option for a special event, when you are doing Phase 2, is to go for the fat options. Eating out in restaurants, hotels or at friends' houses you will hardly ever be offered whole-meal carbohydrates. You are likely, however, to be offered meat, fish, cheese, butter and other fat options. Hence don't eat any carbohydrates that are offered (bread, potatoes and so on) and fill up on the prawn cocktail, steak, salad, cheese, cream sauces and so on and you will not have to cheat at all.

WHEN do you eat?

Eat whenever you want but you really should try to get into the habit of eating three main meals a day and only snacking in between if you are genuinely hungry. There has been a lot of diet advice in recent years that you should 'graze' – eat little and often. Now that you know that insulin is the fattening hormone you know that the fewer times you raise your blood glucose level during the day the better. If you graze, especially if you graze on low fat foods which are always high carbohydrate foods, then you are causing your body to release insulin on a more regular basis and this is what will make you fat.

HOW much do you eat?

The simple advice is – eat as much as you want. However, please be sensible. You are not tricking me if you eat until you feel sick – I will never know! You are only tricking yourself and you are not being at all nice to yourself. However much you may hate your body and, therefore, yourself, it is time to start being nice to yourself. If you don't, no-one else will. Just as you used to stuff your body, now nourish it with wonderful natural, healthy, unrefined foods.

The key reason that this eating plan works so well is that you will find it almost impossible to overeat. Try eating a pound of bacon and 10 eggs when you can't wash it down with fruit juice or tomato sauce or mop up the eggs with bread. Try bingeing on brown rice and stir-fry vegetables. Try overeating steak and mountains of fresh crunchy salad. Try overeating cheese when you can't have biscuits with them. Try overeating bread with no butter and when the bread is genuine whole-wheat with no refined flour or sugar or other processed ingredients. It will be pretty difficult – believe me.

(A small note on bread by the way – as it is such a delicious and filling food, if you are tolerant to wheat, you may like to invest in a bread maker and make your own. Recipe books come with the machines and you can throw in whole-wheat flour and then add sunflower seeds and other tasty extras to make a really nutritious and yummy loaf. This way you can guarantee that it is free from refined carbohydrates).

WHY do you do this?

Phase 2 is designed:
- To continue to win the war against Candida, Food Intolerance and Hypoglycaemia (and thereby to have continued impact on food cravings).
- To continue the great start made in the 'kick-start' phase but with a more varied eating plan that is easier to stick to and more enjoyable.
- To change your eating habits for ever. To put you off one particular food group long term (refined carbohydrates) and to re-educate your palate that there is a wonderful variety of food out there, which is filling and good for you and hugely tasty.

The rationale behind Phase 2 is really simple and powerful:
Rule 1 – Don't eat refined carbohydrates

This is because when you eat refined carbohydrates your body releases the amount of insulin as if you have eaten the whole food (when you drink apple juice your body thinks you have eaten lots of apples remember?) We must stop this happening for two key reasons:

1) As insulin is the fattening hormone we want our bodies to release the right amount of insulin to mop up the food we have actually eaten, not too much so that the extra is stored as fat. If we eat the whole apple or whole grains i.e. the whole food every time, our bodies should release the right amount of insulin.

2) If we end up with too much insulin, after eating something refined, our blood glucose level will be low, which will make us crave food to get our blood glucose level back to normal. Hence we will have cravings for food – especially refined carbohydrates – which is what has made us overeat and overweight in the first place.

Rule 2 – Don't eat anything that will perpetuate any of the three conditions that you are suffering from.

You crave the foods that feed any of the three conditions that you may be suffering from because Candida, Food Intolerance and Hypoglycaemia all lead to unbelievable food cravings. To lose weight you have to stop the cravings. To stop the cravings you have to get these three conditions back under control.

Rule 3 – Don't eat fat and carbohydrate at the same meal.

This is for two reasons:
1) If fat and carbohydrate are eaten at the same time, the body will get its energy from the carbohydrate and store the fat. As we don't want fat to be stored, we must not eat the two food groups at the same time.

2) The second and less important reason is that the stomach produces acid based juices to digest protein and the juices necessary to digest carbohydrate are alkaline. If you eat carbohydrate with protein you are mixing acid juices with alkaline juices and they cancel each other out. Then neither the carbohydrate nor the protein gets digested.

HOW will you feel?

You will feel fantastic! You will not be hungry. You really will not be hungry. You will be free from cravings. You will be eating real, healthy foods which will be nourishing your body and giving you energy like you've not had for years. You can eat both carbohydrate and fat (just not at the same time) so you should not feel deprived. You will be able to eat out and dine in, snack and lose weight, at the same time as keeping your busy lifestyle.

Not only are you eating healthy foods but you are simultaneously avoiding refined carbohydrates, which are unhealthy foods. Hence you are eating the goodies and avoiding the baddies. Most importantly you are avoiding sugar, which is just empty calories, with no nutrients, as we discovered in Chapter 4.

Sugar contains no nutrients, and other refined carbohydrates have had most of their goodness removed in the refining. Hence you will be doing your body so many favours by choosing whole-meal carbohydrates over refined ones, i.e.
- More fibre,
- More nutrients,
- More energy released over a longer period of time,
- Less strain on the pancreas.

In Phase 3 you will be able to choose whether or not you want to eat refined carbohydrates again. It will be interesting to see what choice you make!

Top tips for healthy eating:

There are only three rules in Phase 2 and these are by far and away the most important things to take out of this book. Following just these three rules can change your eating and weight long term. There are, however, some other things that you can do to optimise your health and the way in which you eat. If you do any of these already, well done – keep it up. If not, you may like to try to add another one each month but only when Rules 1-3 are completely second nature to you.

The other good things that you can do are:

1) Don't go hungry.
2) In Phase 3, if you eat fruit with other foods (especially meat and fish), eat the fruit first as it is much quicker to digest and will cause bloating if you eat it afterwards.
3) Drink plenty of water between meals (1.5 litres per day).
4) Don't drink with meals as it doesn't help the digestive process (with the exception of the odd glass of wine – especially red).
5) Don't eat too much saturated fat as it is not as good for you as monounsaturated and polyunsaturated fat.

The tips above are about healthy eating, not weight loss. However, they all have implications for weight loss so they are worth knowing about.

1) If you are hungry you are more likely to crave food as your body will cry out for anything to stop the hunger. So don't go hungry or you will invite hunger pangs and cravings to return.

2) If you eat fruit after other foods, especially meat and fish that take much longer to digest, the fruit gets stuck behind the protein in your digestive tract and this is one of the causes of stomach bloating. This can have an impact on losing weight a) because the fruit is not able to be properly digested by the body and b) because the bloating will make you feel fat and then you may be tempted to eat more – because you already feel fat, so you may as well.

3) If you drink lots of water between meals, your body can rid itself of toxins more easily and all your organs, such as the liver and kidneys, can do their jobs much better. Water also stops hunger pangs because often people are thirsty, not hungry, when they want food. (There is so much water in food that food naturally quenches our thirst – fruits especially). Drinking lots of water also makes you feel energetic and healthy and it is great for your skin and hair. When you feel good you want to make the effort to stick to your eating plan and look good.

4) Drinking at mealtimes floods the body's natural digestive juices and hampers the body's ability to digest the food. The better we digest food, the better it passes through our body so it is important not to do anything to upset the digestive process.

5) As you now know, fat has no impact on insulin and, therefore, does not make you fat. However, there are healthy fats and unhealthy fats. The worst fats are transunsaturated (hydrogenated) fats which are manufactured fats. These you should totally avoid. The next 'not so good' fats are saturated fats so watch how much of these you have to be kind to your body. If you really fancy a pork chop with crackling (about as fatty as you can get) then have it (making sure you only have salad or vegetables with it) because it won't affect your weight. However, the healthier choices are lean meats (especially white meats), any fish and vegetarian alternatives like tofu and quorn. Try to eat as much fish and white meat and as little red meat as possible for optimal health.

KEY POINTS FROM CHAPTER 14

- **Rule 1 – Don't eat refined carbohydrates.**
- **Rule 2 – Don't eat anything that will perpetuate any of the three conditions that you are suffering from.**
- **Rule 3 – Don't eat fat and carbohydrate at the same meal.**
- Follow all of the above for as long as you need to lose weight.
- Eat whenever you want – three meals a day is best but the key thing is not to get hungry.
- Eat as much as you want of everything on the 'allowed' list. Follow the restrictions for Candida and Hypoglycaemia advice.
- Do this because you are following just about the perfect eating plan for all three of Candida, Food Intolerance and Hypoglycaemia.
- During Phase 2 you will feel great, energised, nourished and free from cravings or hunger.

15

PHASE 3

The life-long eating plan

Introduction

This chapter is the nicest gift that I can give anyone who has struggled with their weight, or been out of control with food, at any time in their life. This really is the secret of how to have your cake and eat it. If I had a dollar for every time someone has asked me how I can eat so much, or eat chocolate and ice cream, and stay so slim I could have retired at thirty!

Please note that you should only move onto Phase 3 when you are at your 'natural' weight. The first thing to point out here is that your 'natural' weight may not end up being what you currently expect. There is much evidence that we have a natural weight, which our bodies tend towards. If we put on weight temporarily (e.g. on holiday or during festive seasons) then we will return to our natural weight when we return to normal healthy eating patterns. Similarly if we lose weight during an illness or personal upset we will return to our natural weight when we return to normal healthy eating patterns. I am 5ft 2" and my natural weight seems to be 8st (112lb). I have been below this in recent years, during times of illness or extreme personal stress, and I have gone over this when I have had phases of eating too much chocolate, too often. However, I seem to be able to stay at 8st easily.

You may find that your natural weight is not exactly where you would like it to be. Many people have an 'unnatural' goal for their weight – largely driven by painfully thin models, magazines, peer pressure and unhealthy body images. You may also find that as you exercise and lose weight simultaneously you end up with a toned, athletic shape, rather than a bony, skinny shape which is much healthier and far more attractive.

Hence, please be open minded about your natural weight and for this to be slightly above (or below) your current thinking on your 'ideal' weight. Please note that you may be reading this book when you are actually at your natural weight. You may just want help staying there and you may want a way out of the bingeing and starving, or calorie deprivation, which is probably keeping you at this weight. If this applies to you then you may like to try Phase 2 for a while until you feel free of cravings and in control of your eating and then you can move to Phase 3 quite quickly.

To help you get an idea of where your natural weight will be, on the opposite page is a Body Mass Index chart. If you remember from the opening chapter, BMI is a measure of body fat based on height and weight that applies to both men and women. It is calculated by taking a person's weight in kilograms and dividing this by their height in metres squared.

In the table opposite, find your height in inches along the left hand side and then move your finger along that row until you come to your current weight. Look at the number at the top of that column and that will tell you your **current** BMI. For example, I am 5ft 2in and I weigh 8st (112lb) so I find the row with 62 inches and I am then in the range 109 to 115lb so my BMI is somewhere between 20 and 21. The healthy range is 18.5-24.9 so I am in the middle of the healthy range.

You can then use the chart to see where your weight should be. If you are 5ft 6in (66 inches) then your healthy weight will be somewhere in the range 118-148lb. This is a large range but it allows for both genders and for all different frame sizes. Your natural weight, remember, will be the weight in this range which you can maintain easily – going above it takes some overeating and going below it happens when you are ill or under stress. We all have a natural weight and you will be delighted when you find yours and realise how much you can eat and still stay at this weight.

The guidelines are:
- A BMI of less than 18.5 is considered "Underweight"
- A BMI of 18.5 - 24.9 is considered "Normal"
- A BMI of 25 - 29.9 is considered "Overweight"
- A BMI of 30 or more is considered "Obese"

Please note that the Body Mass Index (BMI) calculator is a guide only. It takes no account of muscle vs. fat for example. Using the BMI scale, many athletes, and almost all rugby or American Football players, are classified as overweight. Please use your common sense when applying this calculator – if you are an athlete or an ex-athlete you will know if you are a solid human being or a flabby one needing some attention!

BMI (kg/m^2)	19	20	21	22	23	24	25	26	27	28	29	30	35	40
Height (in).	Weight (lb).													
58	91	96	100	105	110	115	119	124	129	134	138	143	167	191
59	94	99	104	109	114	119	124	128	133	138	143	148	173	198
60	97	102	107	112	118	123	128	133	138	143	148	153	179	204
61	100	106	111	116	122	127	132	137	143	148	153	158	185	211
62	104	109	115	120	126	131	136	142	147	153	158	164	191	218
63	107	113	118	124	130	135	141	146	152	158	163	169	197	225
64	110	116	122	128	134	140	145	151	157	163	169	174	204	232
65	114	120	126	132	138	144	150	156	162	168	174	180	210	240
66	118	124	130	136	142	148	155	161	167	173	179	186	216	247
67	121	127	134	140	146	153	159	166	172	178	185	191	223	255
68	125	131	138	144	151	158	164	171	177	184	190	197	230	262
69	128	135	142	149	155	162	169	176	182	189	196	203	236	270
70	132	139	146	153	160	167	174	181	188	195	202	207	243	278
71	136	143	150	157	165	172	179	186	193	200	208	215	250	286
72	140	147	154	162	169	177	184	191	199	206	213	221	258	294
73	144	151	159	166	174	182	189	197	204	212	219	227	265	302
74	148	155	163	171	179	186	194	202	210	218	225	233	272	311
75	152	160	168	176	184	192	200	208	216	224	232	240	279	319
76	156	164	172	180	189	197	205	213	221	230	238	246	287	328

Body weight in pounds according to height and body mass index.

WHAT can you eat & drink/not eat or drink in Phase 3 (in brief)?

You really can eat what you want **almost** when you want. This will be called 'cheating'. The key thing is to make sure that the cravings don't return and here is how you achieve this:

1) Don't 'cheat' too much
2) Don't 'cheat' too often
3) Be alert and stay in control

HOW long is Phase 3 (in brief)?

For the rest of your life! This is the way to stay at your natural weight and to eat what you want, to the limit of what you can get away with.

WHEN do you eat (in brief)?

When you are hungry. As with previous advice, you should ideally eat three main meals a day with snacks in between only if you are genuinely hungry.

HOW much do you eat (in brief)?

As much as you want but you will find some tips on cheating in the detailed sections below.

WHY do you do this (in brief)?

You overeat when all you want is to be slim because of food cravings. Your goal in Phase 1 was to attack the causes of the foods cravings. Your goal in Phase 2 was to eliminate the food cravings. Your goal in Phase 3 is to make sure you stay in control so that the cravings don't return. If the cravings don't return you will not be a food addict and you will be able to enjoy a bit of what you fancy when you fancy it.

HOW will you feel (in brief)?

Like a bird let out of a cage! Like the person who has discovered DNA (the secret of life) and the rest of the world hasn't yet realised. Like you can finally be in control of your eating and your weight without depriving yourself of treats for the rest of your life.

Let's go into each of these in more detail:

WHAT can you eat & drink/not eat or drink in Phase 3?

When you end the weight loss plan you can eat anything that you want. That probably bears restating – when you no longer want to/need to lose weight you can eat anything that you want. Chocolate, ice cream, cakes, biscuits, pasta – whatever. However, what you will realise is that whereas before you only avoided certain foods in an attempt to lose weight, you may now choose to avoid certain foods in a desire to feel well. You will get to the stage when you are at a weight you are happy with and you will be able to control your eating as your cravings will have disappeared and you will, therefore, have the choice about what you want to eat. You will be experiencing the following:

- you will no longer crave food,
- you will feel healthy and free from the many physical and emotional symptoms which were described in Part 3,
- you will be eating to live rather than living to eat,
- you will have more energy and zest for life than probably ever before,
- you will be enjoying a wide variety of healthy and nourishing foods.

The ideal eating plan for Phase 3 is to keep rule number one from Phase 2 – don't eat refined carbohydrates – and that alone. Your health will not suffer at all if you never eat another refined carbohydrate again in your life. Hopefully having tasted the nutty flavour and filling texture of brown rice you will never want to return to white rice. Hopefully sugar free multi-grain, whole-meal bread will be your natural choice over white bread any day. There is less difference between whole-meal and white pasta but hopefully the brown variety too will remain your natural choice. You can stick with the Phase 2 eating plan for life and you will live very healthily for doing so. However, if we return to the key attributes of a workable diet in the introduction to Part 4, there may well be reasons for eating refined carbohydrates, on occasions, when your eating and weight are under control. For some people the thought of never eating chocolate or ice-cream again is just too much to think about. You truly will get to the point where you can live without chocolate but it is understandable to think that not everyone will want to do this.

Phase 3 is all about guidelines and the bottom line is to **be alert and stay in control**! You will be armed with a huge amount of knowledge as you set off on a new phase of freedom. You won't eat cartons of Haagen-Dazs and M&M's and not understand why. You will be alert for the three conditions that lead to food cravings and you will be able to nip them in the bud the minute that they reappear.

147

Candida is probably the toughest to keep under control because of the rate at which yeast multiplies. You may start eating refined carbohydrates again and get away with it for days, weeks or even months and then, one day, your cravings will be back as strong as ever and the yeast will have been fed back out of control. One of the best ways to avoid this is to keep your immune system strong. Take a vitamin & mineral supplement every day, take extra vitamin C at the first sign of a cold (a sure sign of a lowered immune system), keep your life balanced and full of things that you enjoy and you will keep the best defence possible against Candida. Avoid antibiotics unless your life is threatened. Avoid hormones and steroids wherever possible.

Food Intolerance is a bit easier to spot – as soon as you become intolerant to a food, you will start to crave it. Watch out for any food that you start to eat every day and stop it immediately. If you start eating a particular food daily or even more than once a day, you are right on the edge of a new intolerance so cut back before the cravings return. Be extra alert for food families (these are covered in Chapter 17). If you find you are eating porridge for breakfast, wholegrain salad sandwiches for lunch and whole-wheat pasta for dinner and are starting to find that you are craving some or all of even these healthy foods, you could have (re)developed a Food Intolerance to wheat. Porridge, bread and pasta are all in the same food family. If you find you are quite quickly becoming susceptible to new cravings then try to rotate the food families that you consume, as Chapter 17 will illustrate.

Hypoglycaemia is easier still to spot – some people get so in tune with their bodies that they know, for example, apples are fine but bananas are too sweet for them. You can't go wrong with meat, fish, tofu, quorn, eggs, dairy and vegetables as far as Hypoglycaemia is concerned, but as soon as you eat higher carbohydrate foods (even fruits and grains) you may find that your blood glucose level is upset. Watch out for a sudden high (energy rush) followed by a low (energy dip) as this is one of the quickest and most obvious indications that Hypoglycaemia is present.

So, here is the secret to having your cake and eating it. The guidelines for Phase 3 are:

1) Don't 'cheat' too much
2) Don't 'cheat' too often
3) Be alert and stay in control

Number 1 says don't 'cheat' too much – eat a chocolate bar if you fancy one but don't eat ten! Eat a dessert if you want one but try to avoid refined carbohydrates in the rest of the meal. Remember your mentality will be changed so you won't think, if you eat a bag of crisps, *"I've blown the day, I may as well eat what I want."* There are no 'good' days and 'bad' days – you are in Phase 3 now, happy with your weight, so you can eat what you want **almost** when you want. You may choose to eat ice cream but you won't choose to eat a three litre tub. Number 1 is, therefore, about the **quantity** of the refined carbohydrates that you eat.

Number 2 says don't 'cheat' too often. Have a dessert for a special occasion, but just not every day. Eat confectionery if you want to, but not every day. Have a blow out at a dinner party or a wedding but just don't do it every day. Number 2 is, therefore, about the **frequency** with which you eat refined carbohydrates. Try to stick to the rules in Phase 2 as often as possible and then cheat on special occasions, or when you really fancy something.

Number 3, as explained above, is about you having the knowledge and the skills to control your cravings and, therefore, to control your eating and your weight. Get to know what works for you like the back of your hand. You may get it wrong the first time and you may find that the cravings return strong and fast. Don't panic. Get straight back on Phase 1 for five days then Phase 2 for however long it takes to get back in control and then learn from the experience. (You may find you can just go back to Phase 2 for a few days and the cravings may subside as quickly as they arrived and you can get back in control easily).

When you learn from the experience ask yourself some questions – Were you cheating too much (quantity)? Were you cheating too often (frequency)? I bet you were more than half aware that you were starting to become quite attached to a particular food or foods and, therefore, you should have cut back earlier as this was the first sign of cravings. Be really honest with yourself next time and as soon as you think you **need** something rather than **want** something, avoid that food, like the plague, for at least five days.

Your entire goal, with eating, from now on is to stay in control of cravings. Cravings make you overeat when all you want is to be slim. You now know how to overcome the cravings. Phase 3 is about making sure that you control them, rather than that they control you, for life.

HOW long is Phase 3?

For the rest of your life! This is the way to stay at your natural weight and to eat what you want to the limit of what you can get away with. What you are really doing is following the three rules in Phase 2 but with the freedom to cheat not too much and not too often so that you stay in control of cravings for ever.

WHEN do you eat?

When you are hungry. Ideally three main meals a day with snacks in between only if you are genuinely hungry. The key point in Phase 3 is that you should limit the number of times you make your body release insulin – especially more insulin than is needed as will happen if you cheat. Hence, if you really fancy a box of chocolates, you are much better off eating the whole box at once than you are having one or two, here and there, throughout the day. If you eat a whole box of chocolates, your body won't recognise the food so it will pump out a response to the sweetness. If you eat the whole box in less than an hour, your body will have one sugar rush to respond to. If you eat the whole box throughout the day, your pancreas will be on continual alert and you will be on a roller coaster of blood glucose highs and lows for hours.

You may realise that this is totally contrary to a lot of the eating advice that has come out recently. We have been advised to 'graze', to 'eat little and often' and to keep our 'blood glucose level constantly topped up'. As you now know, insulin is the fattening hormone and the chance of getting just the right amount released every time, to mop up whatever we have eaten, is very small. We are better off, therefore, not putting constant strain on this delicate mechanism by grazing and asking it to pump out insulin every couple of hours.

HOW much do you eat?

As much as you want but you will find some top tips for advanced cheating below!

WHY do you do this?

You overeat, when all you want is to be slim, because of food cravings. Your goal in Phase 1 was to attack the causes of the food cravings. Your goal in Phase 2 was to eliminate the food cravings. Your goal in Phase 3 is to make sure you stay in control so that the cravings don't return. If the cravings don't return you will not be a food addict and you will be able to enjoy a bit of what you fancy when you fancy it.

Remember the goals of Phase 3:
- To put you back in control of your eating by giving you long term control over food cravings.
- To enable you to eat, without cravings, for life.

- To enable you to eat whatever you want **almost** whenever you want but with you managing the outcome.

HOW will you feel?

You really can feel liberated and empowered in a way you may find hard to imagine right now. Just think how you would feel if you could do the following and stay at your natural weight:

- Never feel hungry and know that you need never feel hungry again.
- Know that you need never go on a fad diet again or count calories or count carbohydrates or count anything.
- Have a box of Belgian chocolates for lunch one day – because you really fancy one.
- Have steak, seafood, pasta, cheese and desserts as things that you can eat regularly because you know the 'rules'.
- Have lunch out and eat tomatoes & mozzarella with olive oil for starter; a delicious creamy, cheesy dish for main course; and then strawberries and cream for dessert. And this isn't even cheating!
- Go to a dinner party, skip the bread and carbohydrates, eat any fat and protein put in front of you, indulge in a portion of the hosts' real French chocolate mousse for dessert, and have everyone wondering where you put it all.

I can give these as real examples because this is how I can now really enjoy food and stay slim, which is what has led to so many comments from friends and colleagues. (As a vegetarian, I skip the steak and seafood, however).

Psychologically, the feelings that come from true freedom from food addiction are incredible:
- Freedom from food obsession,
- Freedom to get on with your life and to hardly think about food from when you wake until when you sleep,
- Freedom to accept and enjoy social invitations and any food that may be there,
- Freedom from guilt, fear, self-loathing and feeling like a failure,
- Freedom from diets and fresh starts,
- Freedom from time wasted because all your energy and ambition is being channelled into eating or not eating,
- Freedom from hunger and overeating hangovers,

And finally,
- The chance to have just one size of clothes in your wardrobe and
- The chance to live, not to exist!

Top tips for cheating!

The basics are really worth repeating – don't cheat too much, don't cheat too often and be alert and stay in control. There are, however, some other great tips that you may like to take on board to become a real cheating connoisseur.

Cheat all at once.
As was advised earlier in this chapter, if you want a box of chocolates eat the box but don't eat one or two chocolates throughout the day. Remember, you are trying to minimise the number of times your pancreas is asked to release insulin.

Have a strategy for getting your blood glucose level back to normal.
If you eat a refined carbohydrate, your body will almost certainly release too much insulin and this will make your blood glucose level fall below what it was before you ate the refined carbohydrate. Your body will then demand food to get your blood glucose level back to normal. This is the time when you are most at risk of craving another refined carbohydrate. Hence, anticipate that this will happen and have something healthy to hand when you feel your blood glucose level drop. This can be a piece of fruit or a whole-meal cereal bar – any whole food which will encourage your blood glucose level to return to normal naturally.

Eat as few ingredients as possible.
The fewer processed ingredients you can attack your body with the better. If you really fancy a bag of crisps/chips then have a bag, but pick the one that has the simple ingredients potatoes, vegetable oil and salt. There are some packets of crisps/chips which have more than one hundred ingredients in them. (The ingredients in a well known global brand of crisps/chips, for example, are: dried potatoes with citric acid, monoglycerides or sodium phosphate; vegetable oil; corn meal; wheat starch; maltodextrin; water; salt; seasoning; spices; flavouring; acetic acid; malic acid; sodium acetate; sodium citrate; mono & diglycerides and dextrose!) Please don't ever be that nasty to your body.

If you want ice cream then have Haagen-Dazs vanilla which has (in order) fresh cream, skimmed milk, sugar, egg yolk and natural vanilla flavouring and tastes as good as ice cream can possibly get. Don't pick the carton with more ingredients than you can recognise let alone remember!

Don't eat your normal meal AND cheat.
If you are going to have a box of chocolates for lunch then make that your lunch. Don't have your steak & salad as well, as your body will just store the fat in the steak when you eat carbohydrates.

Don't waste cheating.
If you are going out for dinner with friends don't start on the crisps and nuts before dinner – you know you'll eat them all as soon as you start so don't even have one. Save the indulgence for the lovely food your hosts have prepared and eat what you really want during the meal. Ditto, when eating out in restaurants don't eat the white bread at the start of the meal and fill yourself up on something that isn't even that tasty. Save your cheating for the real food and enjoy something really special from the menu instead.

Never forget that insulin is the fattening hormone.
Carbohydrates stimulate the production of insulin, the fattening hormone, but so does caffeine. You may like to return to full caffeine coffee and (diet) cola in Phase 3 but this must be counted as cheating. Every time you have caffeine, you stimulate the production of insulin. If this is really how you want to use your cheating then do so. (I prefer chocolate myself!) Cheating connoisseurs never forget that the key to cheating is to minimise the production of insulin.

Get to know your body.
Really get to know your body, exactly what you want, how much you can get away with and how you will feel when you do cheat. Make informed choices and if a clear head and a great night's sleep are more important to you than a sugar induced stupor then make the best choice for you. If you want that sugar, however, then…

Have what you want, what you really, really want.
To misquote the Spice Girls. If you want chocolate, get the best that you can find and afford. Don't settle for a confectionery bar bought from the petrol/gas station, which is more sugar than chocolate. Buy some Belgian chocolates and indulge. Keep them all to yourself, enjoy every one and feel the joy of eating something knowing you are in control of your eating.

Just because you can cheat doesn't mean you have to.
This eating plan lets you eat all the foods that are healthy and nutritious – fruits, salads, vegetables, whole grains, animal and vegetable protein. You will not miss out on anything by not eating refined carbohydrates again so if you don't have any urge to 'cheat' then don't.

KEY POINTS FROM CHAPTER 15

- **Don't cheat too much**
- **Don't cheat too often**
- **Be alert & stay in control**
- You overeat when all you want is to be slim because of food cravings. Your goal in Phase 1 was to attack the causes of the foods cravings. Your goal in Phase 2 was to eliminate the food cravings. Your goal in Phase 3 is to make sure you stay in control, so that the cravings don't return. If the cravings don't return you will not be a food addict and you will be able to enjoy a bit of what you fancy when you fancy it.

16

KEEP TAKING THE TABLETS

Vitamins, Minerals and Nutrition

In some of the recommended reading, for Candida in particular, there are substantial sections on supplements to take for optimal health. Many involve taking tablets at various times throughout the day, some before meals, some with meals and some after. There are oils or liquids to drink as well with some programmes. As the whole idea of this eating plan is that it must be workable and practical I do not propose to recommend such measures.

The only advice in this chapter is to visit a reputable health store and get a good multi vitamin and mineral tablet that works for you. Take advice from the assistants if need be as I have always found them to be most knowledgeable and helpful. There are some 'mega' dose vitamin and mineral tablets and you may think that these will be ideal. However, these tend to be the size of little fingers and many people find them difficult to swallow. I have also found them to be too strong for my small frame and I have felt nauseous and even had itchy skin after taking one. There are some all-in-ones that are not 'mega' and they are easier to take and easier to tolerate. I favour a chewable tablet as I find it easier still to take and it seems to digest easily. The choice is yours.

There are three reasons for advising you to take a multi vitamin and mineral tablet every day:

1) When you read this chapter and understand how important each vitamin and mineral is to your body, the foods that they are found in and in what quantities, you may wonder how we could ever get all the nutrients we need. Taking one tablet, therefore, is like an insurance policy – we will make sure that we get at least the Recommended Daily Allowance of these essential nutrients and then there will be nothing missing for our nutritional health.

2) Our bodies, in their infinite wisdom, will do whatever they can to get us to consume any vitamin and mineral that it is missing. Hence, if there is something missing in our food intake, our bodies will crave

the food that will give us that nutrient. However, our response to cravings is generally not that sophisticated so we don't know that the body is asking for selenium for example and, therefore, wants us to eat kidneys. We may just find that we are craving something and we then eat all sorts of rubbish to try to satisfy that craving.

3) The final, although much less important, reason is that it can't do you any harm. There have been scare stories about taking mega doses of one vitamin daily over a long period of time but one regular vitamin & mineral tablet on a daily basis is not going to cause harm and is likely to do much good.

The single other thing that you can do, which will be fantastic for your health, is to take Essential Fatty Acids as they can be quite difficult to get from your food intake. Remember in Chapter 5 we talked about Omega 6 and Omega 3 oils which are crucial for our health and well-being? Omega 6 oils are found in seeds and their oils – hemp, pumpkin, sunflower, sesame, walnut, soya bean and wheat germ. Omega 3 oils come from linseed, hemp and pumpkin seeds/oils and also oily fish such as mackerel, tuna, salmon and herrings. Unless you eat a lot of seeds and oily fish you will do yourself a great deal of good by buying a reputable source of Essential Fatty Acids when you visit your health food shop. I have a tablespoon of Essential Oils each morning (it tastes OK on its own or you can use it as a salad dressing). You can also buy capsules, which are more convenient if you are travelling. Either way, this is a small step that you can take towards better energy and great looking skin, nails and hair.

VITAMINS
The word vitamin is based upon the term *"vita"* meaning life. There are three criteria that a substance must satisfy to be called a vitamin:

1) the substance must be supplied by what we eat,
2) deficiency of the substance must cause symptoms or disease,
3) those symptoms or diseases are cured only with the relevant substance (vitamin).

There are vitamins A, lots of B vitamins, C, D, E, H (Biotin) and K. Folic acid and niacin are also vitamins which form part of the Vitamin B group. Let us see what they are, what they do, how much we need, where we get them from, what happens if we don't get enough and how we know if we are not getting enough...

Notation
- mg = milligrams
- µg = micrograms = 3.33 IU's (International Units)

VITAMIN A:
What is it?
Vitamin A is a fat soluble vitamin. This means its absorption is improved by consuming fats and oils. It is also known as retinol.

What does it do?
Vitamin A is needed for our sight (remember the saying – carrots help you see in the dark), skin, bones, growth, mucous membranes and to fight infection. It also acts to synthesise protein and acts as an anti-anaemia agent.

How much do I need?
Between 750µg (2500IU)-2250µg (7500IU) per day.

Where do I get it from?
Halibut liver oil (60,000µg per 100g), liver (18,000µg per 100g), butter (750µg per 100g), cheese (385µg per 100g), eggs (140µg per 100g).

What if I don't get enough?
Deficiency in Vitamin A can lead to night blindness, kidney stones, defective teeth & gums, increased susceptibility to infections and rough, dry, scaly skin.

How do I know if I am not getting enough?
Deficiency symptoms include dry eyes, poor sight, burning and itching eyes, poor hair quality, poor scalp quality, scaly skin & scalp and respiratory infections.

VITAMIN B:
We often refer to B Vitamins as being part of "*B Complex.*" This is the mixture of B Vitamins that tends to occur in foods. There are eight members of the Vitamin B Complex. These are:
B1
B2
B3 (niacin)
B5 (pantothenic acid)
B6
B12
Biotin (Vitamin H) (This has a separate entry below the B Vitamins).

Folic Acid (This also has a separate entry).

What are they?

B1 is a water soluble vitamin. It is also known as thiamin(e) and aneurin(e).

B2 is a water soluble vitamin. It is also known as riboflavin(e) and lactoflavin(e).

B3 is a water soluble vitamin. It is also known as niacin.

B5 is a water soluble vitamin. It is also known as pantothenic acid.

B6 is a water soluble vitamin. It is also known as pyridoxine.

B12 is a water soluble vitamin. It is also known as cobalamine.

What do they do?

B1 converts glucose into energy in muscles and nerves.

B2 converts protein, fat and glucose into energy. It is needed to repair and maintain body tissues and mucous membranes.

B3 (niacin) produces energy from glucose, fat and protein. It maintains healthy skin, nerves, brain, tongue and digestive system.

B5 is involved in the production of energy and anti-stress hormones. It controls fat metabolism and helps the formation of antibodies.

B6 helps us metabolise amino acids. It is needed for blood and nerve health, for energy production and it acts as an anti-depressant and anti-allergen.

B12 is needed as the basis of all body cells.

How much do I need?

B1 – approximately 1.5mg daily.

B2 – at least 1.7mg daily.

B3 – between 19mg and 3g daily. Exceeding 3g daily can lead to depression, liver damage, face flushing, dry skin, diarrhoea and nausea.

B5 – at least 10mg daily. No excess problems have been reported.

B6 – at least 2mg daily but not to exceed 200mg daily.

B12 – at least 3µg daily.

Where do I get them from?

B1 – Dried brewers yeast (15.6mg per 100g), yeast extract (3.1mg per 100g), brown rice (2.9mg per 100g), nuts 0.9mg per 100g), pork (0.9mg per 100g), oats (0.6mg per 100g).

B2 – Yeast extract (11mg per 100g), dried brewers yeast (4.3mg per 100g), liver (2.5mg per 100g), eggs (0.47mg per 100g), cheese (0.35mg per 100g), yoghurt (0.26mg per 100g).

B3 – Yeast extract (67mg per 100g), dried brewers yeast (38mg per 100g), nuts (21mg per 100g), chicken (11.5mg per 100g), meat & oily fish (10.5mg per 100g), whole grains (8mg per 100g).

B5 – dried brewers yeast (9.5mg per 100g), pigs liver (6.5mg per 100g), yeast extract (3.8mg per 100g), nuts (2.7mg per 100g), eggs (1.8mg per 100g), poultry (1.2mg per 100g).

B6 – Dried brewers yeast (4.2mg per 100g), yeast extract (1.3mg per 100g), oats (0.75mg per 100g), bananas (0.51mg per 100g), nuts (0.5mg per 100g), brown rice (0.42mg per 100g).

B12 – Pig's liver (25µg per 100g), pig's kidney (14µg per 100g), oily fish (5µg per 100g), beef & lamb & eggs & white fish (2µg per 100g). This is only found in animal foods and, therefore, needs to be taken as a supplement by vegans.

What if I don't get enough?
Deficiency in Vitamin B1 can lead to beriberi but this is rare in the western world.

Deficiency in Vitamin B2 can lead to mouth ulcers, gastric ulcers and eye ulceration.

Deficiency in Vitamin B3 (niacin) can lead to pellagra. This is a disease which causes skin conditions, nausea and vomiting, inflamed digestive tract and depression.

Deficiency in Vitamin B5 can lead to rheumatoid arthritis or allergic skins reactions.

Deficiency in Vitamin B6 can lead to premenstrual tension, kidney stones and depression.

Deficiency in Vitamin B12 can lead to anaemia.

How do I know if I am not getting enough?
Deficiency symptoms of B1 include fatigue, muscle weakness, constipation, irritability, depression, poor memory, lack of concentration and tingling in feet.

Deficiency symptoms of B2 include bloodshot eyes, gritty eyes, tired eyes that are sensitive to light, cracks and sores in corners of mouth, trembling, insomnia and dizziness.

Deficiency symptoms of B3 include dermatitis (skin condition), diarrhoea and dementia.

Deficiency symptoms of B5 include stomach pain, fatigue, insomnia, depression and headaches.

Deficiency symptoms of B6 include splitting of lips, depression, breast tenderness, puffy ankles & fingers and scaly skin on face.

Deficiency symptoms of B12 include sore tongue, menstrual disorders and typical symptoms of anaemia.

BIOTIN/VITAMIN H:
What is it?
Vitamin H is a water soluble vitamin. It is more commonly known as biotin and is a member of the vitamin B complex.

What does it do?
Vitamin H/Biotin is needed for energy production, maintaining healthy skin, hair, nerves and bone marrow.

How much do I need?
At least 300 µg per day.

Where do I get it from?
Dried brewers yeast (80µg per 100g), pig's kidney (32µg per 100g), yeast extract (27µg per 100g), eggs (25µg per 100g), whole grains (20µg per 100g), corn (6µg per 100g).

What if I don't get enough?
Deficiency in Vitamin H/Biotin can lead to fatigue and depression.

How do I know if I am not getting enough?
Deficiency symptoms include fatigue, depression, nausea, smooth pale tongue, hair loss and muscular pains.

FOLIC ACID:
What is it?
Folic Acid is a water soluble vitamin. It is a member of the Vitamin B complex.

What does it do?
Folic Acid is needed for blood formation and to build up resistance to infection.

How much do I need?
Between 400µg-15mg daily. Exceeding 15mg on a regular basis can lead to nausea, flatulence, stomach bloating and sleep disturbances.

Where do I get it from?
Dried brewer's yeast (2400µg per 100g), Soy flour (430µg per 100g), nuts (110µg per 100g), green vegetables (90µg per 100g), pulses & whole grains (80µg per 100g).

What if I don't get enough?
Deficiency in Folic Acid can lead to spina bifida, premature birth, abortion and other birth related complications.

How do I know if I am not getting enough?
Deficiency symptoms include weakness, fatigue, breathlessness, irritability, forgetfulness and mental confusion.

VITAMIN C:
What is it?
Vitamin C is a water soluble vitamin. It is also known as ascorbic acid.

What does it do?
Vitamin C is needed to resist infection, to control blood cholesterol levels and to enable iron to be absorbed into our bodies.

How much do I need?
At least 60mg per day. It is regarded as a safe vitamin and no serious problems have been reported with very high intake. If you take too much the body will get rid of it in your faeces and it can cause loose bowel movements or even diarrhoea if taken in excessive quantities. Nutritionists often advise finding your 'poo tolerant level of Vitamin C'! This means taking Vitamin C in quantities just below that which makes you go to the toilet. This is generally seen as the level of Vitamin C that your body can tolerate and, therefore, needs. You will find that your need for Vitamin C increases when you are fighting an infection. It is recommended to take 1-2g daily as soon as you develop a cold for example.

Where do I get it from?
Brussels sprouts (90mg per 100g), citrus fruits (50-80mg per 100g), cabbage (60mg per 100g), all other fruits and vegetables (20-40mg per 100g).

What if I don't get enough?
Deficiency in Vitamin C can lead to scurvy, which is what afflicted many sailors when they were at sea and away from fresh fruits and vegetables for a long time.

How do I know if I am not getting enough?
Deficiency symptoms include weakness, muscle pains, irritability, bleeding gums, gingivitis (inflammation of the gums) and nose bleeds.

VITAMIN D:

What is it?

Vitamin D is a fat soluble vitamin. It is also known as the sunshine vitamin as we get it from sunlight. We also get Vitamin D from foods of animal origin.

What does it do?

Vitamin D promotes the absorption of calcium and phosphate from food.

How much do I need?

10μg (400IU) per day. This amount should not be regularly exceeded as it is the most toxic of all vitamins. Excess intake can cause nausea, thirst, vomiting, head pain and typical symptoms of sun stroke.

Where do I get it from?

Cod liver oil (210μg per 100g), mackerel (18μg per 100g), tinned salmon (12.5μg per 100g) and eggs (1.75 μg per 100g).

What if I don't get enough?

Deficiency in Vitamin D can lead to tooth decay, muscular weakness and a softening of the bones (rickets) which can cause bone fractures or poor healing of fractures.

How do I know if I am not getting enough?

Deficiency symptoms include bone pain, muscular weakness, muscle spasms and brittle bones.

VITAMIN E:

What is it?

Vitamin E is a fat soluble vitamin.

What does it do?

Vitamin E reduces the oxygen needs of the muscles, acts as an anti-blood clotting agent and maintains healthy blood vessels.

How much do I need?

Approximately 30mg per day, but this amount should not be regularly exceeded as it can lead to nausea, diarrhoea and muscle weakness.

Where do I get it from?
Cod liver oil (60mg per 100g), roasted peanuts (12mg per 100g), shrimps (6.6mg per 100g), olive oil (4.6mg per 100g), green vegetables (2.3mg per 100g), pulses (1.7mg per 100g).

What if I don't get enough?
Deficiency in Vitamin E can lead to dry skin, poor muscular & circulatory function, the death of red blood cells and an inability of the white blood cells to resist infection.

How do I know if I am not getting enough?
Deficiency symptoms include low energy, lethargy, apathy, lack of concentration, irritability and a decreased sexual interest.

VITAMIN K:
What is it?
Vitamin K is a fat soluble vitamin.

What does it do?
Vitamin K's sole function is to control blood clotting.

How much do I need?
Approximately 500-1000µg daily.

Where do I get it from?
Cauliflower (3600µg per 100g), Brussels sprouts & broccoli (800µg per 100g), lettuce (700µg per 100g), spinach (600µg per 100g), cabbage & tomatoes (400µg per 100g).

What if I don't get enough?
Deficiency in Vitamin K can lead to excessive bleeding in the stomach.

How do I know if I am not getting enough?
Deficiency symptoms include diarrhoea.

VITAMIN	NEEDED FOR?	DAILY NEED	BEST SOURCES?
A	Sight, skin, bones, growth, anaemia	750-2250µg 2500IU7500IU	Halibut liver oil, liver, butter, cheese, eggs
B1	Energy conversion	1.5mg	Dried brewers yeast, yeast extract, brown rice, nuts
B2	Energy conversion	1.7mg	Dried brewers yeast, yeast extract, liver, eggs, cheese
B3 (Niacin)	Energy conversion, skin, nerves, brain	19mg-3g	Dried brewers yeast, yeast extract, nuts, meat & fish
B5	Controls fat metabolism	10mg	Dried brewers yeast, yeast extract, pigs liver, nuts
B6	Blood, nerves, mental health	2-200mg	Dried brewers yeast, yeast extract, oats, bananas, nuts
B12	The basis of all body cells	3µg	Pigs liver & kidney, oily fish, meat, eggs – only animal foods
Biotin	Energy conversion, skin, hair, nerves & bone marrow	300µg	Dried brewers yeast, yeast eggs, whole grains, corn
Folic Acid	Blood formation & resistance to infection	400µg-15mg	Dried brewers yeast, soy flour, nuts, green vegetables, pulses
C	To resist infection, control cholesterol & absorb iron	60mg-3g	Fruits & vegetables
D	Bones & muscles	10µg (400IU)	Cod liver oil, oily fish, eggs, sunshine
E	Healthy blood & anti-blood clotting	30mg	Cod liver oil, peanuts, olive oil, green vegetables
K	Controls blood clotting	500-1000µg	Green & other vegetables

MINERALS

The word mineral literally means "*mined from the earth*." There are four types of minerals:

1) Metallic elements that are present in large quantities in the body and in what we eat (like calcium, magnesium, potassium).

2) Non metallic elements that are present in large quantities in the body and in what we eat (like carbon, phosphorus, sulphur). Please note that only phosphorus is defined below as this is the only element of these three that we need to consume in food.

3) Metallic elements present in very small quantities in the body and in what we eat (like chromium, copper, iron, zinc).

4) Non metallic elements present in very small quantities in the body and in what we eat (like iodine, selenium).

These are all very important for our health and well-being. Let us now look at minerals in exactly the same way that we looked at vitamins:

CALCIUM:
What is it?
Calcium is a metallic element found in bones and teeth.

What does it do?
Calcium builds and maintains healthy bones and teeth. It controls the functions of nerves and muscles, it controls the contraction of the heart and other muscles, it assists in the process of blood clotting, it controls blood cholesterol levels and it helps with the absorption of Vitamin B12.

How much do I need?
Approximately 500-1000mg per day. Quantities significantly in excess of this should not be taken on a regular basis, particularly at the same time as high doses of Vitamin D, as the two together can cause deposits of calcium in the kidneys, heart and other soft tissues.

Where do I get it from?
Hard cheeses (1200mg per 100g), soft cheeses (725mg per 100g), tinned fish (400mg per 100g), nuts (250mg per 100g), pulses (150mg per 100g), milk (120mg per 100g).

What if I don't get enough?
Deficiency in calcium can lead to rickets or osteoporosis.

How do I know if I am not getting enough?
Deficiency symptoms include bone pain, muscle weakness and slow healing of bone fractures.

CHROMIUM:
What is it?
Chromium is a metallic element.

What does it do?
Chromium is a really interesting mineral for us and our interest in insulin and overeating. Chromium acts as a Glucose Tolerance Factor (GTF). This means it controls the blood glucose level by making sure the muscles and organs can use the glucose effectively. It stimulates the burning of glucose for energy. It controls blood cholesterol levels, reduces fat levels in the blood and suppresses hunger symptoms by acting on the part of the brain that makes us feel full.

How much do I need?
Approximately 200μg per day. If there is one supplement that you should consider taking, in addition to your multi vitamin and mineral, chromium is the one to take. This can help regulate your blood glucose level and help you feel less hungry and would be a great supplement to take.

Where do I get it from?
Egg yolks (183μg per 100g), dried brewers yeast (117μg per 100g), beef (57μg per 100g), hard cheese (56μg per 100g), liver (55μg per 100g) and vegetables (21μg per 100g).

What if I don't get enough?
Deficiency in chromium can lead to increased blood cholesterol levels and impaired blood glucose balance. It has even been shown that deficiency of chromium led to a condition resembling diabetes in experiments with rats.

How do I know if I am not getting enough?
Symptoms of chromium deficiency are very similar to symptoms of Hypoglycaemia – irritability, mental confusion, weakness, depression, shaky hands, thirst and hunger and so on.

COPPER:
What is it?
Copper is a metallic element.

What does it do?
Copper is necessary for the formation of healthy bones, for developing resistance to infection and for skin and hair.

How much do I need?
At least 2mg daily. The good news is that this is generally achievable with an average daily food intake.

Where do I get it from?
Liver (8mg per 100g), shell fish (7.6mg per 100g), dried brewers yeast (3.3mg per 100g), olives (1.6mg per 100g), nuts (1.4mg per 100g), pulses (0.8mg per 100g). Much of the copper we consume doesn't come from the food we eat but from copper kettles, copper water pipes and other copper containers.

What if I don't get enough?
Deficiency in copper can lead to anaemia and rheumatoid arthritis.

How do I know if I am not getting enough?
Deficiency symptoms include anaemia, water retention, irritability, brittle bones, dull hair and loss of sense of taste.

IODINE:
What is it?
Iodine is a non metallic element.

What does it do?
Iodine is crucial to the functioning of our thyroid hormones. The thyroid hormones control the level of metabolism in the body. They are necessary for converting food into energy and how we use that energy.

How much do I need?
Approximately 200µg per day but this amount should not be substantially exceeded on a regular basis as it can be toxic in very large quantities.

Where do I get it from?
Dried kelp is an amazing source of iodine with 535μg per gram. haddock (659μg per 100g), whiting (up to 360μg per 100g). Fruits, vegetables, cereals and meats also provide small amounts.

What if I don't get enough?
Deficiency in iodine can lead to an under active thyroid or cretinism. Iodine deficiency is seen as an important world health problem as hundreds or millions of people suffer from diseases related to iodine deficiency.

How do I know if I am not getting enough?
Deficiency symptoms include apathy, drowsiness, sensitivity to cold, lethargy, muscle weakness, weight gain and rough & dry skin.

IRON:
What is it?
Iron is a metallic element.

What does it do?
Iron acts as the oxygen carrier in red blood cells. It helps develop resistance to infection.

How much do I need?
Approximately 15-18mg per day. This amount should not be significantly exceeded on a regular basis as iron can be toxic in very large quantities.

Where do I get it from?
Dried brewers yeast (20mg per 100g), liver (13mg per 100g), kidney (12mg per 100g), cocoa powder (11mg per 100g), parsley (8mg per 100g), dried fruits – especially apricots (6mg per 100g). Please note that your cravings for chocolate, which contains a lot of cocoa, may in fact be your body crying out for iron, especially at the time of the month for women.

What if I don't get enough?
Deficiency in iron can lead to anaemia.

How do I know if I am not getting enough?
Deficiency symptoms include those of anaemia – tiredness, pale skin, breathlessness, dizziness, headaches, insomnia and palpitations.

MAGNESIUM:
What is it?
Magnesium is a metallic element.

What does it do?
Magnesium plays a part in many body functions including energy production, cell replication, body cell growth, repair and maintenance of body cells.

How much do I need?
Approximately 400mg per day. Quantities significantly in excess of this should not be taken on a regular basis as excess amounts of magnesium can lead to flushing of the skin, thirst, low blood pressure and upset stomachs.

Where do I get it from?
Soya beans (300mg per 100g), nuts (250mg per 100g), dried brewers yeast (230mg per 100g), whole-meal flour (140mg per 100g), brown rice (120mg per 100g), sea foods (80mg per 100g), dried fruits (80mg per 100g), bananas (40mg per 100g). A very good source of magnesium is also bottled water – especially hard water.

What if I don't get enough?
Deficiency in magnesium has been linked to heart disease because death rates from heart attacks are higher in soft water areas worldwide.

How do I know if I am not getting enough?
Deficiency symptoms include weakness, tiredness, nervousness, involuntary twitches, low blood glucose and painful swallowing.

MANGANESE:
What is it?
Manganese is a metallic element and is essential for human beings.

What does it do?
Manganese is very important for growth in the human body. It helps maintain the nervous system, it is important for our body cells and sex hormones.

How much do I need?
Approximately 2.5-5mg per day.

Where do I get it from?
Cereals (5mg per 100g), whole-meal bread (4mg per 100g), nuts (3.5mg per 100g), pulses (2mg per 100g), fruit (1mg per 100g).

What if I don't get enough?
Deficiency in manganese has been found in the blood of people suffering from diabetes, heart disease, schizophrenia, rheumatoid arthritis and muscle wasting. The link between manganese and these conditions is not totally clear but the association is widely recognised.

How do I know if I am not getting enough?
There are no specific deficiency symptoms related to manganese.

PHOSPHORUS:
What is it?
Phosphorus is a non metallic element which is naturally present in the body and hence deficiency is highly unlikely.

What does it do?
Phosphorus is needed for healthy bones and teeth. It is needed in the production of energy, in the burning of glucose for energy, as an activator for the Vitamin B Complex and to help absorb many components of food.

How much do I need?
Approximately 1.5-2g per day are normally consumed daily so deficiency is unlikely. However, phosphorus does need Vitamin D in order to be absorbed by the body.

Where do I get it from?
Yeast extract (1900mg per 100g), dried brewers yeast (1750mg per 100g), dried skimmed milk (950mg per 100g), wheat germ (900mg per 100g), canned fish & hard cheeses (500mg per 100g), cereals (300mg per 100g).

What if I don't get enough?
Deficiency in phosphorus can lead to anaemia or subnormal white blood cells which can lead to infections.

How do I know if I am not getting enough?
Deficiency symptoms include weakness, bone pain, joint stiffness, irritability, tremor, mental confusion. Please remember, however, deficiency is rare – if you are showing signs of phosphorus deficiency, it

may well be Vitamin D deficiency is the real problem as poor levels of Vitamin D will harm the absorption of phosphorus.

POTASSIUM:
What is it?
Potassium is a metallic element. It is present in all human beings. A person weighing 65kg has about 140g of potassium in their body.

What does it do?
Potassium plays a crucial role in maintaining water balance within the body. It is also involved in energy production and it has important roles to play in keeping our body cells healthy.

How much do I need?
Between 2 and 6g daily. Diarrhoea, abuse of laxatives, fasting, unhealthy diets, anorexia and many other conditions can all cause potassium deficiency.

Where do I get it from?
Soy flour (around 2g per 100g), dried fruits (anything up to 1.8g per 100g), salad vegetables & nuts (up to 1g per 100g), fruit (up to 450mg per 100g), brown rice (200mg per 100g).

What if I don't get enough?
Deficiency in potassium can lead to paralysis or collapse in the extreme.

How do I know if I am not getting enough?
Deficiency symptoms include vomiting, bloating stomach, muscle weakness, 'pins & needles' and drowsiness & confusion.

SELENIUM:
What is it?
Selenium is a non metallic element.

What does it do?
Selenium is needed for normal liver function, it helps fight infection, it keeps hair, skin, eyes and heart healthy. It acts as an anti-inflammatory and helps to protect against toxic substances.

How much do I need?
Approximately 200µg per day. Quantities significantly in excess of this should not be taken on a regular basis as it can lead to hair, nail and skin weakness.

Where do I get it from?
Kidneys & liver (40µg per 100g), fish & shellfish (30µg per 100g), whole grains & cereals (12µg per 100g).

What if I don't get enough?
Deficiency in selenium can lead to keshan disease (a congestive heart disease).

How do I know if I am not getting enough?
Deficiency symptoms include hair, nail & skin problems and heart problems.

ZINC:
What is it?
Zinc is a metallic element.

What does it do?
Zinc is crucial for growth in a human being. It is also important to insulin activity and it helps maintain a healthy liver.

How much do I need?
Approximately 15-20mg per day. Zinc is generally seen as a very safe mineral to take as a supplement. Tests have been done on levels of 150mg consumed daily and have not been found to have toxic effects.

Where do I get it from?
Oysters are by far the best source (70mg per 100g), liver (8mg per 100g), dried brewers yeast (8mg per 100g), shellfish (5mg per 100g), meat & hard cheese (4mg per 100g), canned fish (3mg per 100g).

What if I don't get enough?
Deficiency in zinc can cause sexual problems in men. Deficiency can also cause growth failure and impaired sense of taste in both genders.

How do I know if I am not getting enough?
Deficiency symptoms include eczema, hair loss, mental apathy, impotence, post natal depression and loss of taste and smell.

SUMMARY (MINERALS)

MINERAL	NEEDED FOR?	DAILY NEED	BEST SOURCES?
Calcium	Bones & teeth	500-1000mg	Milk, cheese, tinned fish, nuts, pulses
Chromium	Controls blood glucose level	200µg	Egg yolks, dried brewers yeast, beef, cheese, liver
Copper	Bones, skin, hair, to resist infection	2mg	Liver, shell fish, dried brewers yeast, olives. Also copper pipes & containers
Iodine	Thyroid function	200µg	Kelp, haddock, whiting & small amounts in other fish
Iron	Oxygen carrier in red blood cells	15-18mg	Dried brewers yeast, liver, kidney, cocoa, dried fruits
Magnesium	Energy production, body growth & repair	400mg	Soya beans, dried brewers yeast, nuts, whole grains
Manganese	Growth & nervous system	2.5-5mg	Whole grains, nuts, pulses
Phosphorus	Bones & teeth, activates the B complex for energy	1.5-2g	Yeast extract, dried brewers yeast, canned fish
Potassium	Energy production, water balance, body cell health	2-6g	Soy flour, dried fruits, salads, vegetables, nuts, fruit, brown rice
Selenium	Liver, heart, hair, skin, eyes, fights infection	200µg	Kidneys & liver, fish & shellfish, whole grains
Zinc	Growth, insulin balance	15-20mg	Oysters, liver, dried brewers yeast, shellfish, meat, cheese, fish

173

What else can I read if I want to know more?

"Thorsons Complete Guide to Vitamins and Minerals" by Leonard Mervyn (1986)
"The Optimum Nutrition Bible" by Patrick Holford (1998)
"Boost your immune system" by Patrick Holford (1998)

KEY POINTS FROM CHAPTER 16

- The most important note to take away from this chapter is the marvel of the human body! When you read all about the vitamins and minerals needed for your body to function, hopefully it will shock you into giving your body what it needs.
- Every single food source for every single vitamin and mineral is a natural food. Everything that we need can be found in real foods – meat, fish, eggs, milk, vegetables, grains, nuts, fruits and so on. We have no need whatsoever for additives and manufactured ingredients.
- Two of the most common symptoms of vitamin and mineral deficiency are tiredness and irritability. If you are feeling tired and not your usual jovial self, it could well be that you are not eating a key vitamin or mineral that your body needs.
- Take a multi vitamin and mineral tablet daily just to make sure that you get at least the Recommended Daily Amount of each nutrient. Seriously consider taking a good source of Essential Fatty Acids as well and possibly a chromium supplement if you really want to do the best for your health.
- Eat as wide a variety of foods as possible to make sure that you get as many nutrients as possible from your food.
- Start nourishing your body and being nice to it – if you don't, no one else will. From now on good days mean those when you nourish yourself with vitamins and minerals and bad days are days when you binge or starve and aren't nice to yourself.

17

WHERE'S THE SUGAR?

Food families & where to find hidden ingredients

What are food families?

Foods are grouped into 'food families', to indicate which foods have similar characteristics and origins to each other. Food families are of interest for both Candida and Food Intolerance as it is important to know which foods are related when you are trying to avoid foods which are harming your health. You may avoid bread in an attempt to avoid wheat without realising that pasta is in the wheat family too. Hence, if you carry on eating pasta, when you are trying to overcome your craving for bread, you will just be feeding your craving in a related way and you will continue to crave both bread and pasta.

Below is a list of food families. A main food group, such as "meat, fish & dairy", is broken down into smaller groups of foods that are deemed to be in the same 'food family'. The 'Cattle' food family, for example, has lamb and beef amongst other things but rabbit is in a food family on its own.

Meat , Fish & Dairy:

CATTLE	Beef, veal, lamb, goat, milk, cheese, yoghurt
PIG	Pork, ham, bacon
DEER	Venison
RABBIT	Rabbit
PHEASANT	Chicken, pheasant, quail, partridge
GROUSE	Grouse, turkey, guinea fowl
DUCK	Duck, goose

EGGS	Are very similar in the proteins that they contain and are, therefore, in a separate category.
FISH	Are just about all in one family. If people are sensitive to all fish, this is generally food **allergy,** rather than Food Intolerance and can show sensitivity to

parvalbumin, which is a protein in all fish in the main group eaten (trout, salmon, cod, haddock etc).

Some people are sensitive to 'shellfish' and not other fish, but this generally also implies food allergy rather than Food Intolerance. Shellfish include crab, lobster, crayfish, shrimp, prawn etc.

Fruit & Nuts:

ROSE -	PLUM	Plum, prune, cherry, nectarine, almond, apricot, peach
ROSE -	BERRIES	Blackberry, strawberry, raspberry, rosehip
ROSE -	APPLE	Apple, pear
CITRUS		Orange, grapefruit, lemon, tangerine clementine, lime, kumquats
BANANA		In a family on its own (with plantain)
PAPAYA		On its own
GRAPE		Grape, raisins, sultanas
BILBERRY		Blueberry, cranberry
PINEAPPLE		On its own
GOURD		Melon, cucumber, squash, pumpkin
CASHEW		Cashew, pistachio, mango
WALNUT		Walnuts, pecans
PALM		Coconut, dates, palm oil
CURRANT		Blackcurrant, redcurrant, gooseberry

Grains:

GRASS -	POOIDAE	Wheat, rye, oats, barley
GRASS -	PANICOIDEAE	Maize (corn), sugar cane
GRASS -	BAMBUSOIDEAE	Rice
BUCKWHEAT		On its own

Herbs & Vegetables:

BEAN & PEA	All beans, peas, alfalfa, lentils, peanuts, liquorish, senna, soya beans, chickpeas, carob and mange tout.
CABBAGE	Mustard, cabbage, cauliflower, broccoli, Brussels sprouts, turnips, horseradish, radish, cress, watercress and swede.
DAISY	Lettuce, endive, chicory, artichoke, chamomile and salsify.
ONION	Asparagus, onion, garlic, leek, shallot and chives.
CARROT	Parsley, parsnip, carrot, celery, fennel, coriander, celeriac, aniseed, dill, cumin and coriander.

POTATO	Potato, tomato, aubergine/eggplant, peppers, chilli, paprika and tobacco!
SPINACH	Beetroot, sugar beet and spinach.
CUCUMBER	Melon,cucumber, squash, pumpkin and courgette/zucchini.
FUNGI	Mushrooms and yeast.
MINT	Mint, basil, oregano, rosemary, sage and thyme.

Where can we find the most common Food Intolerance substances?

Dairy Products:
Foods which always, or invariably, contain dairy products include milk, cheese, yoghurt, ice cream, cream, butter, creamy pasta sauces, cakes and biscuits.

Ingredients you may see listed, which are invariably dairy products, are casenin, lactalbumin, lactose and whey.

Wheat:
Foods which always, or invariably, contain wheat include bread, crisp breads (unless specifically rice based – rye is in the same family as wheat), pasta, cereal, flour, pastry, biscuits and cakes.

Ingredients you may see listed, which are invariably wheat based, are cereal protein, cereal binder, cereal starch, starch, edible starch and modified starch.

Corn:
Foods which always, or invariably, contain corn include cornflakes, corn based cereals, corn on the cob, sweet corn and polenta.

Ingredients you may see listed, which are invariably corn based, are corn meal, corn starch, corn syrup, edible starch and glucose syrup.

Eggs:
Foods which always, or invariably, contain eggs include omelettes, pasta and cakes. Biscuits often contain egg based ingredients

Ingredients you may see listed, which are invariably egg based, are lethicin and ovalbumin.

Soy:
Foods which always, or invariably, contain soy include **tofu**, soy sauce, soy flour and soya bean oil. Soy products are derived from soya beans.

Ingredients you may see listed, which are invariably soy based, are lethicin and vegetable protein.

Peanuts:

Foods which always, or invariably, contain peanuts include Snickers bars, peanut butter, some cakes & biscuits. Because of genuine nut food allergies, nuts are almost always clearly identified on food packaging and in food outlets. However, these packaging alerts normally just say 'may contain nuts' not which nuts may be present.

Sugar:

Foods which always, or invariably, contain sugar include confectionery, biscuits, ice cream, crisp breads (many), bread (most), cereal (almost all), soups (many), salad dressings (many), pasta and cooking sauces (most), crisps (many) and prepared meals (most).

Ingredients you may see listed, which are invariably sugar, are dextrose, maltose, glucose, sucrose, lactose (milk sugar), maltose, fructose and glucose syrup – anything ended in "*ose*" should be suspected as a sugar ingredient. Other ingredients to avoid are treacle, syrup, golden syrup and honey as they are refined sugars with other names.

Hopefully you will develop the view that it is far better to eat natural ingredients than packaged foods, which have up to one hundred ingredients for you to check. Why buy a pasta sauce, which almost certainly contains wheat and sugar if not dairy products as well, when you can fry some onions and garlic (great to kill off Candida), add some tomatoes (tinned with nothing added or fresh) and a few mixed herbs and you have a quick, tasty and very healthy pasta sauce. You can even make a big batch and freeze it for future use. (There is a great recipe in Part 10 for a five minute tomato pasta sauce).

Rotation Eating Plans:

For some people with extreme Food Intolerance, advice is given to follow, what is called a Rotation Eating Plan. This means that you rotate the foods you eat so that you don't eat the same foods every day. It generally takes three to four days for a food to work its way fully through our bodies and, therefore, any food which we eat more frequently than this can lead to Food Intolerance. An example Rotation Eating Plan is shown below. I recommend one, which repeats over a weekly basis (a four day plan which then repeats three of the four days) so that you can get into a weekly pattern of 'it's Monday so it must be oats.'

	ANIMAL PROTEIN	VEGETARIAN PROTEIN	GRAINS	FRUIT
MON/FRI	MEAT – Beef, veal, lamb, goat FISH – White fish	Cows milk, Goats milk, Cheese, Yoghurt Lentils	Oats Buckwheat	Apple, pear
TUE/ SAT	MEAT – Chicken, pheasant, quail, rabbit FISH – Oily fish	Quorn Beans Cashews, Pistachios	Brown rice or brown rice pasta	Grapes, Kiwi, Tropical fruits (melon, papaya, mango, pineapple)
WED/SUN	MEAT– Pork, ham, bacon FISH – White fish	Tofu Walnuts, Pecans Chickpeas	Whole-Wheat Pasta Rye Cous-cous	Berries (strawberry, raspberry, blueberry etc), Bananas, Citrus fruits
THUR	MEAT – Turkey, duck, goose, venison FISH – Shellfish	Eggs Quorn	Corn, Polenta Potatoes *	Stone fruits (plum, prune, cherry, nectarine, peach, apricot)

* Potatoes are a vegetable not a grain but they can be eaten in rotation.

Another option is to go for a strict 4 day Rotation Eating Plan but this then means every day will change as you start on a Monday for the first cycle, then Friday for the second cycle then Tuesday for the third and so on. If you do need to follow a Rotation Eating Plan, the one below gives you a choice from each of the food groups on each day of the week. It also gives both animal protein and vegetable protein options each day so that vegetarians can follow it too.

Please note that this is not a totally 'perfect' Rotation Eating Plan as, for example, oats are in the wheat family and are, therefore, eaten just two days after wheat in the above eating plan. However, this is close to perfect and the small variations are for pragmatism – to make sure that you can have as wide a variety of foods as possible each day, to ensure that you get enough to eat. Porridge is also a food that people are rarely intolerant to on its own and it is an excellent food to eat for nutrition and cholesterol (it has been shown to lower cholesterol).

(Polenta, for those of you who haven't come across it, is cornmeal cooked slowly to form quite a 'meaty' texture. It is similar to tofu in texture and very tasty).

The next table shows the meal options for this rotation diet. The V in the table indicates suitable for vegetarians. The R indicates that this recipe is in Part 10.

	BREAKFAST	MAIN MEALS	SNACKS
MON/FRI	Porridge oats with milk or water Natural Live Yoghurt Fruit	-Cauliflower cheese (R, V) -Aubergine dishes (R,V) -Lentil moussaka (R, V) -Cheese & oat biscuits (V) -Steak & salad -Roast lamb, lamb chops -White fish & vegetables -Halibut in cheese sauce	Fruits of the day NLY Milky cappuccinos Oat biscuits Cheese
TUE/ SAT	Tropical fruit platter Fish Rice cereal (sugar free)	-Quorn in tomato sauce (V) -Mushroom risotto (V) -Vegetarian chilli & brown rice (R, V) -Cold brown rice salad (V) -Chicken salad -Roast chicken -Salade Niçoise (R)	Fruits of the day Rice cakes Cashews, pistachios
WED/SUN	Berry compote (R, V) Fresh or baked bananas Bacon & Ham Whole-wheat cereal (sugar free)	-Stir-fry vegetables with tofu (R,V) -Whole-wheat pasta and tomato sauce (R, V) -Cous-cous & chick peas (R, V) -Whole-wheat bread salad sandwich (V) -Pork chops & vegetables -Ham salad -White fish & vegetables/salad	Fruits of the day Smoothies Walnuts, pecans Ryvita crackers
THUR	Stone fruit platter Omelette Fried eggs Scrambled eggs Cornflakes (sugar free)	-Eggs - any style (V) -Quorn or polenta in tomato sauce or baked with vegetables (V) -Baked potato & salad (V) -Turkey roast & vegetables/salad -Shellfish platter & salad	Fruits of the day Hard boiled eggs Dried apricots Corn cakes

KEY POINTS FROM CHAPTER 17

- Foods are grouped into 'food families' to indicate foods which have similar characteristics and origins to each other.

- Food families are of interest for both Candida and Food Intolerance as it is important to know which foods are related when you are trying to avoid foods that are harming your health.

- The most common foods to which people are intolerant in the US are dairy products, wheat, corn, eggs, soy, peanuts and sugar. These ingredients are found in many different forms, in many different products, and you need to be alert. Read ingredient lists very carefully if you are intolerant to any foods.

- A Rotation Eating Plan is an excellent idea for anyone suffering from severe Food Intolerance or for those people who tend to eat the same foods each day and, therefore, develop new intolerances quite quickly. Foods pass through the body within four days, so a Rotation Eating Plan makes sure that you don't exposure yourself to the same foods more frequently than this.

EATING & NUTRITION – A SUMMARY

PHASE 1 – 5 DAYS

- **Do eat** meat, fish, eggs, (tofu – if you are tolerant to soy products), quorn, Natural Live Yoghurt, any salads, any vegetables (except potatoes or mushrooms), some brown rice, herbs & spices, olive oil and butter.
- **Do drink** still or sparkling water, herbal teas, decaffeinated tea or coffee.
- **Don't eat** anything that is not on the list above. No fruit, no wheat or grains (other than brown rice) no white rice, no sugar, no cakes, no biscuits, no confectionery, no cheese, no pickled or processed foods.
- **Don't drink** alcohol, fruit juices, soft drinks, low calorie soft drinks, caffeinated products or milk.

PHASE 2 – AS LONG AS YOU NEED TO LOSE WEIGHT

- **Rule 1** – Don't eat refined carbohydrates.
- **Rule 2** – Don't eat anything that will perpetuate any of the three conditions that you are suffering from.
- **Rule 3** – Don't eat fat and carbohydrate at the same meal.

PHASE 3 – LIFE-LONG

- Don't cheat too much.
- Don't cheat too often.
- Be alert & stay in control.

TOP VITAMIN AND MINERALS TIPS

- Take a multi vitamin & mineral tablet daily
- Ideally take a tablespoon of Essential Fatty Acids and extra Vitamin C daily

(You may like to tear this page out and put it in your wallet).

PART 5

RATIONALISATION
& EXPLANATIONS

DOES MY BUM LOOK BIG IN THIS?

Why are more women than men obese?

The International Union of Nutrition Sciences has published the following statistics on their excellent web site www.iuns.org. The following table shows examples of the prevalence of obesity in adults throughout the world:

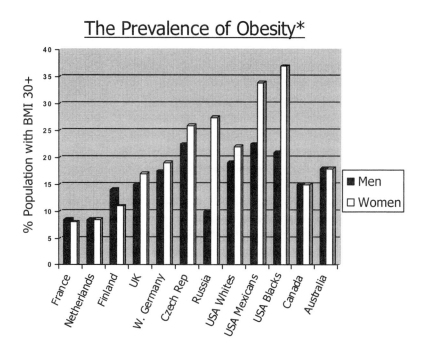

(* All data 2001 or later)

Only in Finland was there a significant result showing more obese men than women. In all other countries the results were either close or obesity in women was significantly higher. Some of the differences are vast.

There are a number of reasons why more women than men are obese:
1) Number one is calorie counting.
   a) More women than men count calories and women also go on more calorie counted diets than men i.e. there are more women calorie counting and they calorie count more often than men. As calorie counting slows down the women's metabolism, the women will then put on weight eating the same amount that they did prior to their first diet. This is how people put on more weight the more they count calories.

   b) Calorie counting then encourages Food Intolerance and/or Candida in a number of different ways:
      - First, calorie counters weaken their immune system by consuming less energy than their body needs and often by consuming fewer vitamins and minerals than their body needs.
      - Secondly, calorie counters often neglect protein foods in favour of lower calorie alternatives, thus denying the body a crucial food group.
      - Thirdly, calorie counters nearly always have a very restricted range of foods, which they eat to the exclusion of all others, simply because these foods are lower in calories than others.
      - Finally, the type of foods which calorie counters eat are often those which feed Candida (such as cottage cheese, fruit, fruit yoghurts, occasional sweet treats and low calorie drinks) or those to which allergies commonly develop (cheese, tomatoes and oranges for example).

2) Women are more susceptible to the conditions that cause cravings – Candida, Food Intolerance and Hypoglycaemia. Candida is markedly more prevalent in women – the mere fact that women buy yeast medication over the counter shows how Candida (yeast overgrowth) is generally a woman's problem. The vagina is an ideal place for Candida to proliferate to a degree that cannot be paralleled in men. Add to this the hormonal upheaval women experience every four weeks, with their monthly cycle, and we have an ideal environment for parasites to take advantage of the immune system. Finally, only women take the contraceptive pill, which Candida thrives on, and women also more often take antibiotics for cystitis and other infections.

All of the theory in this book, therefore, is consistent with the empirical evidence which shows that women world-wide tend to be more obese than men.

KEY POINTS FROM CHAPTER 18

- Globally, more women than men suffer from obesity.
- Calorie counting, Candida, Food Intolerance and Hypoglycaemia are all more prevalent in women than men and, therefore, serve as a useful explanation for why more women than men suffer from obesity.
- The calorie counted foods chosen by women particularly cause Candida, Food Intolerance and Hypoglycaemia.
- The female anatomy is a better breeding ground for Candida than the male's body.

19

FAT BANK ACCOUNTS, SLIM PROGRESS

Why has obesity got worse
as we have 'developed' as nations?

As we noted in the introduction, we started the new millennium with equal numbers of overweight and underfed people, for the first time in human history. The year 2000 registered 1.1 billion overweight people and 1.1 billion underfed people – that is one third of the world's population, literally, stuffed or starving.

Obesity is now, therefore, as big a world issue as malnutrition and starvation. Will we have a Live Aid concert not to save the starving in Africa but to save the obese in the United States? What an unbelievable thought. Why has this happened? There are many reasons:

- Sugar consumption has increased dramatically so that 'civilised' nations now consume approximately a pound and a quarter of sugar per person per week. The calories we get from sugar are not providing nutrients so our bodies still need other foods and liquids to gain the vitamins and minerals we need for our health. Remember sugar also requires nutrients to digest it but it gives none back in return and, therefore, depletes our nutrient reserves. We, therefore, need to eat even more food on top of the sugar we eat to compensate for the nutrients we lose digesting sugar.
- The Calorie myth has much to answer for. Fewer people would be as obese as they are today if they had not slowed their metabolisms over the years with repeated calorie controlled diets.
- Stress and higher paced lives have led to a change in our eating habits. We now favour refined and processed foods that can be eaten quickly. Stress has also affected our health and immune systems which, in turn, has left us more susceptible to Candida, Food Intolerance and Hypoglycaemia.
- Twentieth century drugs – we have introduced a number of drugs into everyday lives in the twentieth century, all of which will have had an impact on our natural health balance and immune systems – antibiotics, hormones, the pill, steroids etc.

The theories in this book explain the increasing prevalence of obesity. Food cravings – driven by dieting, Candida, Food Intolerance and Hypoglycaemia – are at the heart of the widespread increase in obesity...

- Sugar has a direct impact on Candida, Food Intolerance and Hypoglycaemia. It feeds Candida, is commonly craved as part of Food Intolerance and directly affects blood glucose levels. All of these conditions in turn lead to food cravings and obesity.
- Calorie counting, as we have repeatedly shown, can make people fatter in the long term due to the impact that calorie counting has on metabolism and food cravings.
- Stress has a direct impact on Hypoglycaemia as the adrenal glands affect blood glucose stability. Prolonged stress also weakens our immune system which can lead to Candida, Food Intolerance and Hypoglycaemia.
- The drugs which have become more common in the last century have directly contributed to Candida as they have upset the natural balance in our bodies that keep Candida under control.

There are two other factors:
1) In the developed world we exercise considerably less than our predecessors who were active throughout the day. We also exercise less than people in 'underdeveloped' nations. We have so many modern gadgets. We can travel in machines, whereas humans previously went by foot or animal. We can wash with machines, get water from a tap not a well, clean our living areas with gadgets and even change TV channels without moving more than a finger. This has undoubtedly lowered our metabolisms and changed the amount of food we need to survive.

2) At the same time our eating has gone up – we now have more time to eat than we had before (we don't have to spend the morning hunting animals – we can pop into a fast food restaurant and have food whenever we want). We also have more choice than ever to tempt us and more advertising to tell us about all these temptations. We used to eat simple foods such as vegetables, meats, fish and fruit. We now eat processed foods with up to one hundred separate ingredients on the packet.

In summary, food cravings are making people overeat and gain weight and these can be traced to three physical conditions – Candida, Food Intolerance and Hypoglycaemia. All of these conditions were almost unheard of a century ago and, therefore, as they have become more and more widespread, so obesity has increased. The three conditions have dramatically increased in prevalence due to a number of factors – an increased consumption of sugar and refined carbohydrates, wide-spread calorie counting in continued attempts to lose weight, more stressful and higher paced lives, the introduction of drugs such as antibiotics and the pill, a significant change in our eating patterns and a dramatic reduction in our level of exercise.

KEY POINTS FROM CHAPTER 19

- Globally, obesity is now a similar size problem to starvation – both conditions affect approximately one billion people.
- Obesity is only a problem in developed nations where food is in abundance.
- A number of things that are typical of developed nations have contributed to the rise in obesity – calorie counting, increased sugar consumption, stress and modern drugs such as antibiotics. All of these can cause Candida, Food Intolerance and Hypoglycaemia which in turn can cause food cravings, overeating and overweight.

20

ONCE I START I CAN'T STOP

Why do we get into vicious and virtuous circles?

Have you ever noticed how you get into vicious and virtuous circles? You start eating healthily and it goes well for a few days. The more you stick to healthy eating, the easier you find it to stick to. Suddenly things are going well, you feel in control of your eating, you start noticing a difference on the scales and in the way your clothes fit. You feel elated. You are finally back in control of your eating. You feel that you have the power to lose weight and you feel really good. Then what happens? That voice in your head makes an unhelpful suggestion or two – *"why not?"*, *"you can cope"*, *"you haven't binged for ages – you'll be fine with a bit of what you fancy."* So, you have some chocolate, or something else that you normally crave, and then the following happens:

Hypoglycaemia

After eating the craved food your blood glucose, which has been quite stable for days, is suddenly jolted back into the peaks and troughs of Hypoglycaemia. Your blood glucose level rises quickly and gives you a huge high that you may not have had for days. This, however, is then followed by the big trough as your body releases (too much) insulin and your blood glucose level drops lower than it was before. Then the cravings come back big time. Your blood glucose level is so low that your body cries out for any carbohydrate – just to raise your blood glucose level again. That one piece of chocolate or refined carbohydrate suddenly leads to more chocolate and more refined carbohydrates and you are into a full-scale binge.

Food Intolerance

Having stayed off your trigger foods for a few days, you could have a number of reactions after suddenly eating a food to which you are intolerant. A few people experience quite violent and unpleasant symptoms as the body sensibly alerts you to the fact that this is an unwelcome food. In *"Not all in the Mind"* by Dr Richard Mackarness, a situation is described whereby a man, severely intolerant to eggs, avoided them for a period of time and then inadvertently ate them in a cake and literally collapsed after eating them. You may find, if you are quite intolerant to wheat, for example, that you experience quite strong symptoms after eating wheat for the first time in a few days. Symptoms can include severe bloating/abdominal distension, an 'upset' stomach, significant water retention (illustrated by the fact that some people can weigh up to 7lb heavier from one day to the next when they eat a food to which they are intolerant) and a general feeling of being unwell.

Other people can feel significant elation after returning to their addictive substances and they are immediately caught back in the trap of cravings and food addiction. They may still have adverse reactions (water retention is one of the most common) but there is also a psychological well-being which makes it difficult to continue to avoid the offending food(s). Whether you experience positive feelings, or just negative reactions, you will have re-introduced your 'poison' to your body and the cravings will start to return. In the chapter on weight maintenance, where we talk about 'cheating', you will note that you need to be very sensitive to your own susceptibility to cravings.

Candida

The third thing that happens when you eat a food, which you have avoided for some time, is that you may reawaken the Candida overgrowth inside you, which you are unlikely to have killed off with just a few days healthy eating. As soon as you eat yeasty and sugary foods you start to feed the Candida again and your Candida led cravings will rapidly return. So we have the two extremes – the virtuous circle and the vicious circle – and Candida, Food Intolerance and Hypoglycaemia explain why these happen. We assume for the diagram overleaf that healthy eating means avoiding foods that contribute to Candida, Food Intolerance and Hypoglycaemia. The vicious circle is the exact opposite:

VIRTUOUS CIRCLE

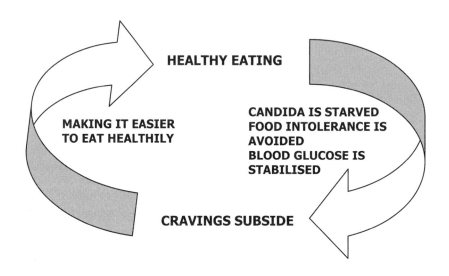

HEALTHY EATING

MAKING IT EASIER
TO EAT HEALTHILY

CANDIDA IS STARVED
FOOD INTOLERANCE IS
AVOIDED
BLOOD GLUCOSE IS
STABILISED

CRAVINGS SUBSIDE

VICIOUS CIRCLE

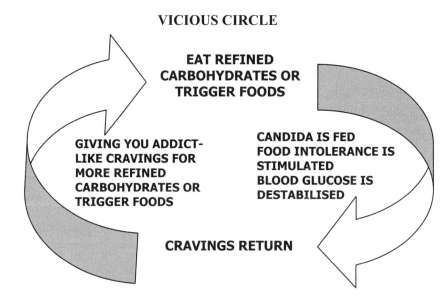

EAT REFINED
CARBOHYDRATES OR
TRIGGER FOODS

GIVING YOU ADDICT-
LIKE CRAVINGS FOR
MORE REFINED
CARBOHYDRATES OR
TRIGGER FOODS

CANDIDA IS FED
FOOD INTOLERANCE IS
STIMULATED
BLOOD GLUCOSE IS
DESTABILISED

CRAVINGS RETURN

In as little as one day, and certainly in no more than three to five days, you can move from a virtuous circle to a vicious circle. The good news is that you can break out of a vicious circle to a virtuous circle in the same amount of time.

You need to get your immune system strong again, free from Candida and Food Intolerance and your blood glucose well under control before you can start to cheat. At the moment, when you can move so quickly from a virtuous circle to a vicious circle, this is a clear indication that your immune system is not strong enough and you need to be free from Candida, Food Intolerance and Hypoglycaemia before you try to cheat. Don't lose heart! You will be able to cheat and there is nothing like savouring the taste of chocolate when you **want** to eat it rather than when you **need** to.

KEY POINTS FROM CHAPTER 20

- It is not coincidental that you get into vicious circles downwards or virtuous circles upwards.
- The more you eat the foods that cause you problems, the more you feed Candida, the more you perpetuate Food Intolerance and the more you upset your blood glucose balance and experience Hypoglycaemia.
- When you avoid the foods that cause you problems, you kill off the Candida, you recover from Food Intolerance and you stabilise your blood glucose level and ease Hypoglycaemia.
- The best bit of news is that you can move from a vicious circle downwards to a virtuous circle upwards in just a few days.

PART 6

PSYCHOLOGICAL FACTORS

21

EAT TO LIVE OR LIVE TO EAT

Why do we eat and why do we overeat?

Emotional reasons for eating and overeating

Having explored the physical reasons for overeating, let us now turn to the emotional reasons. I work as a Human Resources professional and one of the best training courses I have ever attended was with the Australian founders of the Restorative Justice process. Restorative Justice is also known as 'conflict resolution conferencing' and the idea is that people in conflict are brought together to resolve their differences by talking. It works for two reasons:

1) The average human being would rather be in harmony with others than in conflict.
2) The power of the group (mob mentality) will work to help individuals in conflict tend towards harmony.

I mention this because one of the most fascinating parts of the course was about our six basic emotions. We learned on the course how to recognise these emotions, through words and body language, so that we could harness them to achieve group harmony.

We have six basic emotions that we express as human beings. The words in the English language that best describe them are:
- Interest
- Fear
- Surprise
- Distress
- Anger
- Enjoyment

We eat for many reasons and many of these reasons are related to our emotions. The key reason for eating should be to feed our body, to nourish it by giving it the vitamins and minerals that it needs. Our ancestors did tend to eat for this reason and for them food was about survival. They needed enough food to keep warm and to keep starvation and illness away. We seem to eat now for almost any reason other than that we are hungry or require vitamins or minerals. We tend to eat for emotional reasons so let us look at these six basic emotions...

Interest – We do eat out of curiosity. We eat because we want to know what something tastes like. If we have eaten chocolate cake before we want to see what that particular chocolate cake tastes like. Even if we can pretty much guarantee what something will taste like, we still seem to want to eat that substance to see what it will taste like right now in this moment.

Fear – On the course, real fear was one of the most important emotions that could be observed on people's faces, as conflict resolution conferencing could be highly emotional. Human beings tend not to eat when facing genuine fear. The last thing on a hijack victim's mind is food. When experiencing a nasty road rage attack, people are not thinking about food. We do tend to eat, however, when faced with mild and perhaps inappropriate fear. Have you ever been to a supermarket the day before a public holiday? Do we stockpile or do we stockpile?! It is as if we fear running out of food. I have never known anyone die of starvation in the western world over Thanksgiving, Yom Kippur, Christmas or any other celebratory festival. Yet we shop and eat as if this is bound to happen.

This 'fear' of going without food is by no means limited to the handful of days each year that the shops are closed. We fear going without food for even a few hours. How many people eat in the airport terminal because they don't know when their next meal is due? How many people eat the aeroplane food for exactly the same reason – we don't know when we will land, when we will get to our destination, when the next meal will be. Only diabetics need food with this kind of certainly and regularity. The rest of us are eating it a) because it is there and b) because of the bizarre sense of fear of when we will next see food. (My suggestion for the not knowing when the next meal is due is to carry a whole-meal energy bar with you when travelling and then you will always know that you can stave off genuine hunger if you need to).

Surprise – In conflict conferencing, surprise is a fascinating emotion as this is how the real breakthroughs are made. When dawning realisations occur to all parties as to why other people did what they did, the most difficult relationships can turn full circle. In our generally less serious day to day world, surprise is a rare emotion. Think about the last time something really surprised you. When did you last have that wonderful expression on your face that surprise elicits?

With eating it is almost certainly the **lack** of surprise in our daily lives that makes us eat, rather than surprise itself. Lack of surprise is of course boredom. How often do you eat because you are bored? You're in a dull meeting and the lunch sandwiches arrive and you see it as the answer to your prayers. At least now you have something fun to do. You are waiting in a queue, in traffic, to collect the children, for someone to arrive and I bet you think of food way more than even you normally would. You are bored. You are lacking surprise in your life. Take a really honest look at your life at the moment. Is it too mundane? Can you predict how the next week, fortnight, month is going to pan out? Do you have little to look forward to? Do you have nothing that will really surprise or excite you? If this is the case, you will inevitably be driven towards 'comfort eating' as your life lacks the surprise and excitement that we need as human beings and you are using food as a way to fill this void.

Distress – Now we get into a really interesting emotion when it comes to food. Extreme distress is likely to stop people eating. When people suffer bereavement, or the end of a special relationship, they suffer extreme distress and often eat considerably less than they would normally. People have been known to lose pounds after the loss of a family member or divorce. Genuine and extreme distress, like genuine and extreme fear, generally takes away our emotional need for food. Again, as with fear, it is the milder and more regular distress that we suffer day to day that drives us to eat for emotional reasons. Another word for distress is sadness. When we are generally sad, as opposed to the huge trauma of loss, we tend to eat for emotional reasons. We eat to cheer ourselves up. We didn't get the job we wanted, the person we fancy doesn't fancy us, we are feeling low because the dark nights are drawing in, we are just having one of those blue periods in life – this is when we reach for food as a comfort. We literally look to food to cheer us up. The real sadness is that it doesn't work. If food did cheer us up, the world would be a much happier place than it is now.

When we eat, we don't just deal with sadness. A lot of other emotions come into play. We feel the initial high of the food getting into our bodies (or literally the blood glucose level rising in our bodies, as we now understand) but the more we eat the guiltier we feel. The angrier we feel at ourselves, the more disappointed and so on. We feel all kinds of emotions but we rarely feel cheered up, which was the reason for eating in the first place.

Anger – is a fascinating emotion. Entire books have been written about anger and food. There is actually a physical reason why we eat when we are angry. Anger triggers the 'fright, flight, fight' mechanism in our

200

bodies. The anger physically causes adrenalin to be released into the blood, because the body is getting ready to deal with the crisis and to help us 'fight' or 'flight' (run away). The problem is, when we are sitting in our cars and we experience road rage (either ourselves or against us), the fright, flight, fight mechanism works beautifully, the body gets itself ready for the fight or for running away, and yet nothing happens. We rarely confront the other driver so all the adrenalin that was there ready for the battle has nowhere to go. It sits within us instead and we just have to live with the rage. Physically and emotionally we are now heading towards a huge urge to eat. Physically our blood glucose level is just about to drop because the adrenalin rushing around has not been dealt with. Emotionally we have all this rage that has not been dealt with and it turns inwards instead. We feel so angry and yet we have not had a chance to get even. We get even with a box of chocolates or a packet of biscuits instead.

Two inspirational trainers, with whom I had the great pleasure of working, gave me an insight into anger that has had a profound effect on my thinking. Kevin Downey and Brad Waldron, founders of "Oxygen Learning", told me that *"Anger is a pill that you swallow hoping to make someone else ill."* We can lie there at three o'clock in the morning feeling rage towards another person and yet they have absolutely no idea that we are doing this. We are the ones feeling the rage, hoping that they will feel the pain. They don't, we do.

Think about all the times that you eat out of anger or frustration and start getting alert to your emotional reasons for eating. Your partner didn't do what you wanted them to do so you feel angry and turn to food. The children are driving you mad so you eat. Your boss or work colleagues are making you angry so you eat. Your family are making unreasonable demands of you and not considering your needs. Who in fact is suffering for all the anger you are feeling? Not the other people that is for sure. Don't swallow this anger pill, and all the emotional turmoil that goes with it, because it doesn't have the desired effect on the person or situation you are angry with.

Enjoyment – is the final basic emotion that we are exploring in relation to food. This has quite obvious connections with why we eat. We eat when we are sad and we eat when we are happy. Human beings don't seem to need an excuse to eat. Often when we are ecstatically happy we don't eat. When we fall in love, or when our wedding day is approaching, or when we are about to go on a trip of a lifetime, we often feel so happy that we don't eat and people can lose pounds in the early days of a new relationship. However, as we saw with fear and distress, it is only in the extreme of an emotion that we tend not to eat. When we feel moderately happy or content we can turn to food to try to give us even more enjoyment. Once the new relationship has gone past the really exciting first few days or weeks, quite often people put back on the weight that they lost and more. The happy couple have breakfast in bed together, they go out for dinner, they have picnics in the park, they 'spoil' each other with chocolates and other edible gifts and the weight soon goes back on.

We eat when we feel contentment, therefore, and we eat because we think it will give us enjoyment. We eat emotionally for the pleasure we think that food will give us. However, the enjoyment is very short lived. As the saying goes – a minute in the mouth and a lifetime on the hips. We get very brief enjoyment from eating refined carbohydrates in particular as they are so easy to swallow. Nature's own food delights, such as mangos or pineapples, take longer to eat and chew and can, therefore, be even more enjoyable.

We also eat because we think it will make enjoyable experiences even more so. We go to the cinema and we eat ice cream, M&M's and popcorn and wash it down with additive filled fizzy drinks. Does this really make the movie more enjoyable? Does it make us feel good inside? There are so many emotional reasons why we eat that are related to enjoyment. We eat because we are enjoying something or because we think it will make us enjoy that something more.

A final point to make in relation to eating for enjoyment is that, when you are addicted to a particular food, you move quickly from eating that food for enjoyment, to eating it to avoid the opposite of enjoyment, which is what happens when you don't have it. This means that you will no longer feel enjoyment when you eat a food to which you are addicted. However, you will feel bad if you don't eat it because you will have withdrawal symptoms and so you mistakenly think you will feel enjoyment if you do have it. Only when you are no longer addicted to food can you really savour tastes and genuinely enjoy food. Until then, the food is controlling you, rather than the other way round.

We tend to eat, therefore, when we are not experiencing the real extremes of our basic emotions but when we are in that middle band of 'normal' life. However, this means that for the vast majority of our lives, during this normal range, we have emotional drivers to make us eat. We don't seem to need an excuse to eat and yet there are many – boredom, road rage, travel, public holidays and new relationships – anything and everything that happens to us in life seems to have an emotional connection to food. Why is this?

The Impact of Childhood

There is another saying that goes something like "*Show me the child of seven and I will show you the adult.*" This saying states that the child of seven has experienced the vast majority of the development in life that they will go through and, therefore, their preferences, personality traits and behaviour are all determined at this early age. Some people now suggest seven is late and that the final personality is formed in most people as early as the age of three or four. So for any of you with children over seven the argument says that your work is over – there is not much that you can do now to change how your child is going to be in later life. What a thought!

In relation to food, however, it is fascinating to note the messages that we give children and, therefore, the messages that they carry with them throughout life:

- We tell them to eat everything on their plates. This means we are telling them to ignore their own hunger mechanism (which actually works pretty well in children) and to eat whatever **we** have decided to put on their plate.
- We rarely ask them what they want to eat – we decide instead what **we** think they should have and then battle with them to get them to eat it.
- We try to take away the real enjoyment of meal times for children and insist that they behave and don't play with food. Playing with food can be immense fun!
- We tell them not to talk with their mouths full and yet they want to both talk and eat so this causes a conflict.
- We set meal times to suit our busy lives rather than asking them when they are hungry and when they want to eat.
- We tell them off for spilling things and yet they don't do this deliberately and they wish, as much as we do, that it hadn't happened.
- We give food constantly as a reward or to cheer children up (they fall over and we give them sweets, they cry and we give them a cookie). This builds up a life-long connection between eating and feeling better.

We give children all sorts of messages about food that stay with them for life. Look at your own childhood and see how many daft messages you are hanging onto that you should now choose to get rid of as a grown-up.

My personal experience was very profound and I have had to work hard to get rid of my early conditioning. My parents were brought up in war time with food rationing and, therefore, had strong ideas about eating everything on a plate and eating whatever was put in front of you whether you liked it or not. My most vivid childhood memories are not of fun playmates or great things that I did but of constant battles with food and grown-ups. I would spend many afternoons at home in the dining room or kitchen not allowed to leave the table until I had eaten what was in front of me – hungry or not and whether I liked it or not. When I didn't eat it (when, not if) it would come out at the next meal and the next meal until it eventually went bad. I never ate anything that I didn't want to (you can take a horse to water but you can't make it drink) but I certainly went through enough battles making sure that I didn't eat.

The same happened at school. I would spend many an afternoon sat in the dining hall with my uneaten food in front of me watching the clock until 3.35pm when school finished and they couldn't keep me any longer. How stupid and outrageous was that? My mother was a teacher at the same school so she would also know that I was in the dining hall and would continue to be disappointed with me. How disappointed was I with the grown-ups? I didn't know just how disappointed (or angry) I was until I first sought help for an eating disorder.

I learned all my later anorexic behaviour during this time. I learned how to push food around the plate to make it look like I had eaten more than I had. I learned how to sit next to 'Greedy Graham' at school so that I could give him the things I didn't want to eat when the teachers weren't looking (a great win-win). I even spoiled my favourite dungarees as a child by stuffing white broad beans into the pockets, when my parents weren't looking, rather than eating them. I learned how to do other 'magic' tricks like slipping food into hankies unnoticed and all the other things that anorexics do like professionals. I learned my eating disorders as a child.

Eating disorders, as we will see in the next chapter, are about control. When I did become anorexic at sixteen, I was taking control of my life away from the control of grown-ups. One of the most fundamental choices we should have as human beings is what should go into our own bodies. As soon as I was 'allowed' to make more choices about what I wanted to eat and when I wanted to eat I took the ultimate control and hardly ate anything. Trying to control our eating is a euphemism for trying to control our lives. The more out of control we feel in our lives, the more out of control our eating gets. To understand and overcome the emotional reasons for eating we need to be well tuned in to the early messages we received, why we eat and what we really are trying to control.

For any adults reading this, who want to do the best for children, the advice I would offer is to let children do what they want as far as is possible. Clearly they need to eat breakfast by a certain time but they can choose whether to eat before or after they get dressed, for example, and they can choose what they want to eat. This doesn't mean giving them a limitless choice, as this is equally stressful for children, but it does mean giving them more than one choice (which is actually no choice). You can ask them if they want cereal, fruit, yoghurt, eggs, brown toast or a combination of any of those. Better still, from about the age of five, you can put options on the table and the children can help themselves. (The best way to get a picky eater to eat more is to put the food in the middle of the table and then they think it is scarce and they need to compete for it. They soon pile their plates up and eat quickly). When there isn't time pressure, ask them when they want to eat (children will generally tell you when they are hungry) and again give them a few options – pasta, chicken & potatoes, sandwiches – what do you fancy? Then make meal times as enjoyable as possible. Eat with them. Make it OK to spill things (they don't do it deliberately). Make it OK to talk. Make it OK to play, within reason. And, whatever else you do, never insist that they eat everything on their plate and never, ever, keep bringing it back again at the following mealtimes until they do eat it. Hopefully this is a pattern of behaviour from a past generation that parents of today are not still following.

I can hear parents now saying 'this is all very well but how do you get children to eat healthy food'? One of the best ways is to give them only healthy food as the choice and to let them play with it. We have had deli bars at home, since the children have been aged five and seven, where we put all kinds of things on the breakfast bar and they make their own meals. They have whole-wheat bread rolls, oat biscuits, a huge variety of cheese, ham, salami, grapes, tomatoes, fruit and anything else we have in the fridge. They then make their own mustard and salami sandwiches with grapes inside, or cheese, ham and tomato falling out of the roll because there is so much filling. They have a great time and they eat a lot and they enjoy it. It also takes less time in the long run to get all the packets out of the fridge and put them on the table and to get everyone to prepare their own food than it does for you to prepare it and then try to get them to eat what you have prepared.

KEY POINTS FROM CHAPTER 21

- This book is focused on physical reasons for overeating and helping you find a way out of food addiction. However...
- We do eat for emotional reasons and there are six basic emotions which can all 'feed' our eating in a number of ways. These basic emotions are interest, fear, surprise, distress, anger and enjoyment.
- Our emotional reasons for eating and overeating are ingrained in our childhood experiences. You may need to seek help from a good friend or a trained counsellor to try to understand your own 'baggage' that you are carrying round emotionally.
- If you have children of your own, or are a child carer in any way, please do whatever you can to give them a healthy attitude towards food and don't give them some of the destructive messages that you may have been given as a child.

22

FAT IS A HUMANIST ISSUE

Eating disorders and the psychological reasons for overeating

What about eating disorders?

Literature has conventionally considered three types of eating disorder – anorexia, bulimia and compulsive eating.

The medical definition of anorexia is *"loss of appetite"* but this does not provide an adequate definition of anorexia as an eating disorder. Anorexia is the prolonged, deliberate abstention from eating despite probable ravenous hunger. It is a conscious decision not a subconscious reaction to a traumatic incident. It manifests itself in a sudden, rapid weight loss leading to an abnormally low body weight. Amenorrhoea (loss of menstruation) invariably follows in women. The sufferer will feel continually cold even in warm weather and down-like body hair may grow as nature tries to compensate for the lost heat energy. Mentally, anorexia is characterised by a paranoid fear of food and of putting on weight. Interest in food, calories, weight and size is obsessive and the single minded determination to avoid food can make a fundamentally honest person furtive and dishonest, as the anorexic will do anything to avoid eating.

This book is not specifically for anorexics in so far as we are trying to understand overeating, not the opposite. However, it must be noted that anorexics often have periods of uncontrolled eating as part of their disorder and, in general, anorexia is often the prelude to bulimia or compulsive eating. The anorexic mentality will be considered further in this chapter on psychological issues. In addition, regarding physical issues, we will assess how the anorexic's continuous deprivation of food, and hence vitamins and minerals, can lay the grounds for Candida, Food Intolerance and Hypoglycaemia.

The general point to make here is that anorexia seems to have psychological roots, which have been discussed at length by various authors. Anorexia is of more interest to us as an extreme example of how calorie deprivation precedes Candida, Food Intolerance and Hypoglycaemia and how there are physical foundations underlying binge eating disorders.

From the one eating disorder, which features the under-consumption of food, we turn to the two which feature over-consumption of food – bulimia and compulsive eating. The distinction between the two is generally assumed to be that bulimics overeat and then attempt to compensate by taking laxatives and/or being sick and/or starving whilst compulsive eaters overeat without necessarily trying to purge or starve afterwards.

What are the symptoms?

Physically, bulimics tend to be normal or near normal weight whilst compulsive eaters may be considerably overweight. However, as a result of their attempts to purge their binges, bulimics may suffer further physical symptoms – tiredness, stomach disorders, dry skin and hair, amenorrhoea in females (periods having stopped), muscle weakness, headaches, palpitations and tooth decay to name just a few of the many side effects. Vitamin and mineral deficiency inevitably occurs as the absorption of food is disturbed. Psychologically there is little to distinguish bulimics and compulsive eaters from anorexics – all share the same paranoid fear of food and of putting on weight and a complete obsession with food. All overeaters, whether lapsed anorexics, bulimics or compulsive eaters, would identify with some or all of the following descriptions of themselves:

- To be obsessed with, yet terrified of, food.
- To think about food from the minute you wake up until the minute you fall asleep.
- To be terrified of putting on weight.
- To fear social situations where you may not be able to determine what food may be on offer.
- To decline social invitations for this reason.
- To decline social invitations because you want to lose weight before seeing so-and-so again.
- To judge a day purely by the amount of food you have, or have not, consumed, not by what you have done or achieved.
- To be overwhelmed with guilt for eating an apple if you vowed not to eat an apple that day.
- To hate yourself.
- To feel a failure.
- To decline a dinner invitation as you don't intend to eat that day.
- To decline a dinner invitation for the above reason and then stuff yourself for the entire evening instead.
- To make a fresh start each and every day.

- To be utterly demoralised by continuous failure.
- To lose all faith and confidence in yourself.
- To feel that you are having a nightmare that will never end.
- To waste vast amounts of potential because all your energy and ambition is being channelled into eating or not eating.
- To be unable to sleep some nights due to genuine hunger.
- To collapse into a heavy sleep after a binge and to wake the next morning puffy eyed, bloated, hungover and fat.
- To have two wardrobes.
- To not be able to plan ahead because you don't know what weight you will be and hence you won't know if you will even want to attend a social occasion let alone what you will wear.
- To continually set yourself tougher and tougher 'rules' in an attempt to control your behaviour.
- To feel totally out of control nonetheless.
- To hate the lies and deception which accompany food addiction as you try to avoid food or social occasions.
- To want to be open but to feel the world will despise you.
- To put off living until tomorrow *"when I'll be slim."*
- To exist not to live!

Given this fear of food and weight, and the blinding obsession to be slim **which overrides everything else,** why do bulimics and compulsive eaters gorge food? This is the fundamental question, which this book addresses.

This book is, therefore, very relevant to the bulimic or compulsive eater – to anyone who overeats regardless of whether or not they try to purge the binge. This book is saying that whilst psychological factors do have an important part to play in the understanding of eating disorders, there are physical reasons why people overeat which are just as important if not more so.

The physical reasons are (you should know them off by heart by now):

- Calorie counting, which will make anyone with an eating disorder hungry and likely to crave food.
- Candida, which will make sufferers crave yeasty, sugary, vinegar foods.
- Food Intolerance, which will make sufferers crave specific foods or food families.
- Hypoglycaemia, which will make sufferers crave carbohydrates.

Given the abuse anorexics, bulimics and compulsive eaters have given their bodies; they are extremely likely to be candidates for all three of the conditions in this book. Their immune systems will not be in a good state, they will have depleted their bodies of nutrients for some time and they will be very susceptible to Candida, Food Intolerance and Hypoglycaemia.

Anyone with a serious eating disorder, like anorexia or bulimia, should work through this book like any other person prone to overeating as the reasons for the overeating and the conditions being suffered are the same.

Remember, if you overeat, you are not greedy or weak willed. You are an addict just like a smoker or drug addict and you now have the tool kit to go 'cold turkey' on your food addiction and to stop the cravings for ever.

There is another interesting point, before we leave this chapter on eating disorders – bulimia doesn't work. I sat next to a bulimic in an open plan office once and her eating was unbelievably out of control. She also trained for and ran marathons so the punishment she was putting her body through I can only imagine. She openly shared the fact that she made herself sick after eating and yet she was about 20lb overweight and no amount of exercise or starvation had any effect. Here are a few reasons why bulimia (bingeing & starving or bingeing & purging) doesn't work:

- Newton's second law of motion says that for every action there is an equal and opposite reaction. This is not a joke, or a physics lesson, but a way of saying what is definitely true when it comes to eating. Bingeing leads to starving and starving leads to bingeing – the two are definitely connected and the only way out is to stop either one. Stop bingeing and you won't need to starve or stop starving and you won't need to binge.

- Purging only works if you believe the calorie theory. If you make yourself sick after eating you think that the calories won't be absorbed and, therefore, you will lose weight. Wrong! The pancreas knows as soon as you have eaten food and it releases insulin to mop up that food as soon as the taste buds register that you have eaten something. If you throw up the food, the insulin is still there and, worse still, it has no food to mop up so it all gets stored for a rainy day. Not only does this ruin your blood glucose mechanism and make you more susceptible to diabetes, it doesn't stop the production of insulin, which is the fattening hormone.

- Laxatives also won't work for the same reason – the insulin has already been released so all you do is speed up the exit of food from your body and do your intestines a lot of damage in the process. You may feel lighter, having been to the toilet, but there has been no real weight loss.

Eating disorders are laying the body wide open to all of the conditions of Candida, Food Intolerance and Hypoglycaemia. Eating disorders directly and indirectly cause food cravings and the best thing that you can do is to follow the advice in this book, start being nice to your body and get the cravings well under control.

What else can I read if I want to know more?

"Fat is a feminist issue" by Susie Orbach (1978)
"Hunger Strike: Starving amidst Plenty" by Susie Orbach (2001)
"The Monster within: Facing an Eating Disorder" by Cynthia Rowland McClure (2002)

KEY POINTS FROM CHAPTER 22
- Literature has conventionally considered three types of eating disorder – anorexia, bulimia and compulsive eating.
- This book is about overeating whether the overeater purges (bulimia) or not (compulsive eating).
- This book is not about anorexia which is a complex issue much related to control and feeling out of control. However, anorexia is characterised by severe calorie counting and it does lead to a weakened immune system, poor nutritional intake, stress and over - consumption of carbohydrates (relative to protein and fat consumption, not an absolute over-consumption). All of these factors can lead to Candida, Food Intolerance and Hypoglycaemia, which explains why so many anorexics become compulsive or binge eaters despite an immense desire not to eat and to be slim.
- Bulimic efforts to purge food (such as vomiting or taking laxatives) actually don't work as insulin is the fattening hormone and the body responds to the food being eaten whether or not it is purged afterwards.

23

IT'S UP TO YOU!

The most important chapter in this book
(once you are free from addiction)

This is the most important chapter in this book. There is only one person in the world that can make sure you control your eating and that is you. I sincerely hope that this book helps to show you how but, at the end of the day, it is up to you whether or not you choose to do anything about your eating and your weight.

Food Addiction

For as long as you are addicted to food, I firmly believe that you do not have a free choice about when and what you eat. For you to overeat, when all you want is to be slim, there must be something more powerful than your determination working against you. That powerful thing, which you have to overcome to regain your freedom to choose, is addiction. The smoker is a slave to cigarettes – they feel they have to smoke, rather than that they are choosing to smoke. The alcoholic feels powerless in the face of alcohol – they feel that they have to drink rather than that they are choosing to drink. At the moment you give into that food craving you are in the same boat. You are having to eat that particular substance rather than making a free choice. If you were making a free choice you would not eat it because you want so badly to be slim. The fact that at the particular moment that you eat the substance you do want it more than you want to be slim is a fantastic demonstration of just how powerful food addiction is.

The goal of this book is, therefore, to enable you to be free from food addiction. You now know that calorie counting will make you hungry and liable to crave anything just to get some fuel into your tank. You also know that Candida, Food Intolerance and Hypoglycaemia can all give you incredibly powerful food cravings for specific foods or groups of foods. You also know that the good news is that you can free yourself from these intense food cravings in as little as five days. If Candida is a problem for you then it can take a bit longer for food cravings to disappear but, even with Candida, cravings will subside dramatically during the 5 day kick-start eating plan.

When you follow the advice in this book, you **will** get to the point that you are not craving food in general or specific foods. You **will** be free from food addiction and the overwhelming cravings for food that have been sabotaging your eating goals will be gone. This is when it really will be **up to you!**

At this time, when the addiction has gone, you **will** have a choice. You will not have compulsive cravings and you will be free to choose what you eat and when. At this time you need to exercise your freedom to choose on a regular basis. When you are not compulsively craving chocolate, for example, you will have an opportunity to consume chocolate (at any one of hundreds of thousands of retail outlets across the world). You will be able to make a balanced, level headed choice that you will not feel able to make right now. You will be able to weigh up how much you want the chocolate (note the word 'want' not 'need') and what it will do to you if you do have it.

It's up to you

One of the best books ever written, in my humble opinion, is the *"Seven Habits of Highly Effective People"* by Dr Stephen Covey. It has sold over 10 million copies world-wide so I am probably not alone in this view. Dr Covey analysed self-help books over decades of literature for his PhD and came to the conclusion that there were seven key themes that emerged in different formats throughout all the readings. He translated these themes into seven 'habits' and proposed that people who adopted these habits would be highly effective people. (A habit is something we do without thinking. We can have good habits, like cleaning our teeth, or we can have bad habits like biting our nails – both of them we can do, without thinking, on a regular basis). The first habit in Dr Covey's work is *"Be proactive."* This doesn't just mean the opposite of 'be reactive' – it means much more than this. It means take control of your own decisions and actions proactively so that you are always the one who decides what you do.

If you remember back in Chapter 21 we looked at our basic emotions and how we eat for emotional reasons. We talked about anger as one of the basic emotions and how often we get angry and then overeat later. The really powerful result, which comes when a person truly takes control of their actions, is that they know that they can also control their emotions to a great extent. Have you ever found yourself saying 'so and so made me angry'? The reality is that so and so did something and you **chose** to be angry as your response. Now I can hear you screaming at this book already but just stick with me for a while as the readers currently screaming at this book are those with the most to gain by mastering this concept…

The idea behind "*It's up to you*" is that **you cannot control what happens to you in life but you can control how you respond to it**. Viktor Frankl was a Jewish man who survived the Holocaust despite being in four Nazi concentration camps, including Auschwitz from 1942-1945. He suffered the most appalling conditions imaginable and yet he stayed not just sane but content and at peace with himself throughout. Whilst he realised that his captors had control of his body he refused to let them have control of his mind. He decided that his key freedom was that he could choose how he responded to what was happening around him. He could let it destroy him or he could let it make him a better person. He chose the latter. His book about this experience, "*Man's Search for Meaning*", is just one of thirty-two inspirational literary works he went on to write.

You too cannot control what happens to you in life but you can control how you respond to it. There will be times, hopefully few, when real tragedy touches your life and you will feel unimaginable despair, loss and sadness. You will be a healthier person in the long run if you give in to the natural emotions that you will feel at these dreadful times and cry, scream and do whatever you need to do to let your emotions heal you. Advising you to choose your response to situations is not about turning you into a cold and unfeeling robot. It is, however, about getting you to a level of emotional maturity where you **choose** your responses to situations the vast majority of the time. It is also about understanding the times when you will still get angry or frustrated but knowing why you feel that way and why you have made the **choice** to feel that way.

If you think about that last time when you said 'so and so made me angry' think about what they did and why you chose to be angry. Why did you take that anger pill hoping to make the other person feel ill? What did you feeling angry achieve? Getting in touch with our emotions can tell us so much about our overall well-being at any point in time.

When I see someone getting road rage, carving another car up or edging up to the car in front so that another driver can't get in, I always ask myself what stress is happening in their life, at that moment, to make them that way. Be serious, we do not get angry enough to kill another person (road rage has resulted in many deaths in the UK and US) because they overtook us or because they pulled out in front of us. We may be that angry at our partner, family members, children, boss and so on but we are not that angry at the complete stranger whose driving has come to our attention. The other car driver **chose** to wait until the very end of the lane merging sign before pulling in front of you; you **chose** to be angry about this. That is inappropriate anger, so you need to understand what is really making you angry in your life and what you can do about it.

Understanding why you are really feeling certain things is key to conquering overeating for ever. I know now when I want chocolate because I really fancy the taste at that moment as compared to when I am using it as a comfort blanket for an emotion that I am feeling. Or, more accurately, an emotion that I am trying **not** to feel. We use food in a similar way to how alcoholics use alcohol – we use it to escape and numb the emotions that we don't want to cope with in the world. We feel lonely so we eat to cheer ourselves up. It doesn't cheer us up – it just makes us fat **and** lonely. We feel sad so we eat to cheer ourselves up – we then feel fat **and** sad. Talk to a great friend, or a qualified counsellor if need be, but get to the point where you understand why you eat for emotional reasons. This book will help you take away the physical addiction that makes you overeat but you have to work on the emotional bit too.

One of the most powerful feelings that leads people to overeat is very metaphorical. Many of my case studies have talked about a feeling of emptiness which they try to fill with food. *"I go to the fridge"* said one of them, *"I don't know what I am looking for but I still end up eating something."* You will get to the point with this eating plan where you don't need or crave that food but, if you are still feeling empty inside, you are missing something in life and you need to find out what it is, **because it is not food**.

Whose life is this?

The most seriously overweight people often look desperately for a magic wand to make them slim. They want a doctor to staple their stomach or give them liposuction or wire their jaw so that they can't eat. What they are really asking for is for someone else to take control of their eating because they can't control it themselves. How tragic is this? If you are one of those people who wants control taken away, please give some thought to the following:

- What happened in your childhood with food and control to have given you the messages that you have now?
- How is anyone other than you going to be able to do this for you?

Even when some people have their jaws wired, they have been known to liquidise chocolate so that they can still eat it. Who is this cheating? This is like a naughty child stealing cookies from the jar except that it is much more serious. Grown-ups doing similar things are not cheating anyone other than themselves.

The only person who is going to fix your overeating problem is you. This book will show you the physical reasons why you overeat, what is causing your food cravings and it will give you a way out of the addiction that is controlling your life. This book will help you break free from cravings but thereafter it is up to you. You have to choose to do this. You are the one who has to make the difference. You have one life – please don't waste another day of it overeating. Make today the day that you take control and decide – **it really is up to you.**

There are two more things that we are going to look at in this chapter to help you decide it's up to you. The first is something called Neuro Linguistic Programming and the second is the two voices that slimmers have in their heads – the angel telling you to stick to an eating plan and the devil telling you not to…

Neuro Linguistic Programming (NLP)

NLP is the study of how people think and experience the world. As human beings are so individual and subjective, the outcomes of these studies are models of how people tend to behave. From these models, practitioners of NLP can develop techniques for changing behaviour by changing thoughts and beliefs. Here is why changing thoughts and beliefs can be so key to changing behaviour…

The concept of NLP is that for everything that happens there is a belief that is in your head that determines the outcome. This is easy to remember as Action, Belief, Consequence (ABC). Here is an example – if you or I were to come second at the Wimbledon Tennis Championship we would be absolutely over the moon. If Pete Sampras were to come second he would be gutted. What is different? The Action is the same – coming second at Wimbledon – but the Consequence is very different because of the two different Beliefs which come between the Action and the Consequence. Our Belief would be that this would be our life time greatest achievement. Pete Sampras's Belief would be that he had failed to come first.

There are so many examples of where two people experience the same Action only to have a completely different Consequence because of their different Beliefs. Two people survive the same disaster – one of them has a breakdown and the other lives the most fulfilling life possible. The first had the Belief system *"why me?, how can such a bad thing have happened to me?"* The second may think something like *"I am so lucky to be alive; I will live each day as if it were a gift."*

This has really important applications for slimmers because it is not so much the **Action** that is ruining our diets it is our **reaction** to that

216

Action – and this is determined by our thought process, our Belief in other words…

As we have explained, there are physical reasons why binges happen. Once you start eating refined carbohydrates your insulin production and blood glucose level go into a roller coaster mode and you will continue to crave refined carbohydrates, to try to elevate your blood glucose level, whenever it drops below normal. You are also feeding Candida which leads to cravings and you are getting your Food Intolerance fix so you will need more of this soon to stop the withdrawal symptoms. Hence there are strong physical reasons why you binge once you start. However, there are also psychological things going on that we need to be aware of – you need to be alert to the sabotage going on in your mind at the onset of a binge…

No one ever ruined a day's eating with that first mouthful. It is what you do after that first mouthful that ruins the day's eating.

- Let us imagine that you have vowed not to eat breakfast and then hunger takes over and you find yourself having a bowl of sugary cereal or,
- You vowed not to eat chocolate and you find yourself buying a confectionery bar as you get a morning newspaper or,
- You vowed to 'be good' all day but then you settle down to watch TV and suddenly those potato chips are calling to you from the kitchen…

Sounds familiar? So you give in to each of the events above but this doesn't ruin the day's eating. It is what we **believe** next that leads to a binge day. What do we say to ourselves? I've blown it today so I might as well eat what I want and then start afresh tomorrow. We can't be 'good' today so we will be 'bad' today and then 'good' tomorrow. And can you recall the relief and excitement you feel once you have made that decision? You suddenly 'allow' yourself to eat whatever you want. You may even get quite excited at the thought of what you will have. I could salivate at the mere thought of chocolate, miles away from getting my hands on it! How Pavlovian is that? (From Pavlov's dogs that were trained to salivate at the ringing of a bell after food was given every time the bell was rung).

But all of this is our mind playing games. Who decided the good vs. bad rules in the first place? You did! Who decided not to have breakfast? (crazy decision) You did! And it was you, again, who decided that the 'good' day was over. You have to be alert to the things going on in your head which are leading you to overeat. Remember – no one ever blew a diet with the first mouthful – it was what they decided to do next (yes decided) that blew it. You never blew a diet with the first mouthful – it was what **you** decided to do next that blew it!

Let's find a few ways around this thinking:

First of all you don't have 'good' days and 'bad' days any more – or rather you don't have them like you used to. A good day now is a day when you are nice to yourself and your body. A good day is when you nourish your body and feed it with vitamins and minerals and nutritious food. A bad day is when you are nasty to yourself and your body. This is any day when you binge or starve, or count calories, or try to give your body less food than it really needs.

Another idea is to introduce the concept of a weight maintenance day. In your old life you may only have had 'good' days or 'bad' days. In your old world these were days when you lost weight or days when you gained weight. Now you can have neutral days, when you neither gain nor lose weight, but you continue to nourish your body and eat mostly healthy food but you have the freedom to cheat. This is exactly what Phase 3 is about. Ideally you will only do Phase 3 when you are at your natural weight but you can have a Phase 3 day at any time.

If you do eat something you feel you 'shouldn't' have eaten, don't go back to your old style thinking and eat everything except the kitchen sink. Decide to have a Phase 3 day. You won't register lighter on the scales tomorrow but you won't have another couple of pounds to lose that you have just put on today. If you have something you feel you 'shouldn't' then start a weight maintenance/Phase 3 day – don't cheat too much and don't cheat too often. So finish your cheat and then get back on track for the rest of the day. Don't forget to manage the cravings that may come after eating refined carbohydrates and upsetting your blood glucose level. Eat some whole foods to help regulate your blood glucose after eating refined carbohydrates.

OK, back to our ABC's. Remember it is the **Belief** that leads to the bad Consequence not the Action itself. So let us look at some examples of Beliefs that will lead to different Consequences following the same Action. Let us imagine that you have just started Phase 1 and you find yourself eating a cream cake. There are negative and positive Beliefs that can follow and these can either lead to either a negative or positive Consequence/outcome...

NEGATIVE BELIEFS	POSITIVE BELIEFS (Imagine saying these to your best friend)
Black & white thinking – I've totally failed. I've got to have no sweet things whatsoever.	Things are never black and white – there is not perfection or failure and nothing in between. Why am I so harsh on myself? Would I treat a friend like this?
Mental filter – I never manage to stick to a diet, I'm useless and I'll never lose weight.	I can lose weight. Others have done it and so can I. It is up to me. There is no outside force making me break my diet. I did really well yesterday and I deserve congratulations.
Blowing things out of proportion – I've blown it now I may as well eat every cake in the supermarket. I'll never look nice for the wedding/party etc.	One cake doesn't mean I've failed. I've just got to get back on track and not let it lead to more than it has to. I can still look nice for the event – no one notices a couple of pounds anyway.

The negative beliefs will lead to you eating every cream cake in the supermarket (and more).

The positive beliefs will lead to you choosing not to let one slip spoil the day and to return to sensible eating straight away.

The key message from NLP or Action/Belief/Consequence is that your Belief, your reaction to something, determines the Consequence/outcome. If you have one slip up on this eating plan just get straight back on track. Don't beat yourself up. Don't make it worse and don't do any of the following:

- Don't give in to black & white thinking – '*it has to be all or nothing so I've failed.*'
- Don't allow your mental filter to dwell on the negatives and ignore the positives. When you are beating yourself up you are ignoring all the positive things you have done and can do and only concentrating on the negatives. You wouldn't be so nasty to your best friend so don't do the same to yourself.
- Don't blow things out of proportion – '*I've had one small slip so it is the end of the eating plan.*' This is nonsense and you know it. Don't look for excuses to give up.

The Devil & the Angel – The two voices that slimmers have in their head

You know what this bit is about – you want to eat but you want to be slim. You want that cream cake but you want to get into that outfit for the special occasion. We seem to have two voices going on in our heads all the time – the devil and the angel – and, depending on which one wins, we are 'bad' or 'good'.

This section is about how you silence the devil in your head and let the angel win through every time. When you start Phase 1 the devil is going to go wild. It is going to do whatever it can to get you to feed your food addiction. The Candida will physically be crying out to be fed, your Food Intolerance withdrawal symptoms will be begging you to eat your favourite substance and your Hypoglycaemia will be craving refined carbohydrates. As if these physical things are not bad enough, psychologically, you will be telling yourself the following:

1) Start tomorrow – just enjoy that pizza, chocolate, sandwich today – I can be good tomorrow.
2) A slice of pizza, one chocolate bar, one biscuit can't hurt.
3) I deserve it.
4) I feel fine – maybe I don't have all these Candida things after all.
5) Everyone else is eating chocolate, crisps, cakes around me – it's not fair that I can't so I will.
6) I really want that chocolate bar, muffin, tub of ice cream.
7) I'm going to a dinner party tonight – it would be rude not to eat whatever is put in front of me.
8) It shouldn't go to waste (food in the house, children's leftovers etc.).
9) I'm on holiday or I'm in a restaurant – I won't get the chance to eat all of this lovely stuff tomorrow.
10) Why not?!

These and more are definitely going to be in your mind when you start the eating plan so you need to be armed with strategies to overcome them. Here are some suggestions:

1) *Start tomorrow – just enjoy that pizza, chocolate, sandwich today – I can be good tomorrow.*
Every diet starts tomorrow. It's a cliché that tomorrow never comes but clichés are generally true. Every time you say you will start tomorrow you are doing two things:
- You are putting off the day you take control of your eating and, therefore, your life. You are putting off living rather than

existing. You are letting your addiction rule you, rather than ruling your addiction.

- More seriously you are making it even harder to take control with every day that you continue to be ruled by food. Food addiction does not reach a certain level and then plateau. It gets worse and worse the more you feed your addiction. Remember the characteristics of addiction – you need to consume more and more to have the same high and before long you need to consume more and more just to avoid the low – the highs are no longer there. With every day that you delay tackling food addiction it just gets worse. Yes you can start tomorrow – but it will be even tougher to crack tomorrow. **You have to do this sometime so do it now.**

2) *A slice of pizza, one chocolate bar, one biscuit can't do any harm.*
In Phase 1, any and all of the above will do harm. They are all refined carbohydrates and they will all feed your addiction. If you give in on day one you are back to square one. If you give in on day two you have wasted nearly two days – why do it? If you give in on day three you have wasted nearly three days – that's daft. Giving in on day four or five is even worse. Don't give in to these cravings. The whole purpose of this eating plan is to stop cravings because cravings make you overeat and overeating makes you fat. If you give into the cravings you will never get in the position that they can be controlled. All it takes is five days – stick with it, one day at a time and see for yourself.

Eat more of any food that is allowed if necessary to make you so full that you can't give into the cravings. Drink a glass of water every time you feel tempted to eat your favourite foods. **You have to do this sometime so do it now.**

3) *I deserve it.*
No matter how productive or tough a day you have had at work or at leisure you do deserve to be nice to yourself. Eating refined carbohydrates is not being nice to yourself. Giving in to yeast parasites growing inside you is not nice. Eating foods that your body cannot tolerate is not nice and throwing a brick on your pancreas/insulin mechanism is not nice. You deserve so much more than this. You deserve to live not to exist. You deserve to be free from food cravings. You deserve to be nourished and full of nutrients, not stuffed and full of empty calories. You deserve to be in control of your life not controlled by food. You deserve so many things but refined carbohydrates are at the bottom of the list.

4) *I feel fine – maybe I don't have all these Candida things after all.*

Now you are really scraping the barrel. The devil will tell you anything to try to get you to feed the Candida or to eat the foods to which you are addicted. The very fact that you want these foods so badly says that you are addicted to them. If you really can take them or leave them, then leave them.

If you are overweight, then you are overeating. If you are overeating despite desperately wanting to be slim, you are doing this because you are addicted to food. This is what cravings and food addiction are all about.

Be really honest with yourself – you are a food addict and you have to go cold turkey on your problem foods for at least five days before you can start to break free from your addiction.

5) *Everyone else is eating chocolate, crisps, cakes around me – it's not fair that I can't, so I will.*

Stop being a spoilt child. Life isn't fair – if you haven't learned that by now then you need to watch some videos on famine in Africa or war in Asia. Those people eating what you want to eat are probably food addicts too, chances are that they are overweight; chances are that they don't know why and would give anything not to be. You have the knowledge and tool kit to be slim – to free yourself from food cravings, but you literally want to have your cake and eat it. In Phase 1 and 2 you cannot have your cake and eat it. You need to stop eating cake (and other refined carbohydrates) to get your eating back in control and to get to your natural weight. When you are there you can have the things that people around you are eating. You will be able to stay slim and cheat, not too much and not too often, provided you stay alert and in control.

Just stick with it for now, free yourself from cravings and then you may find you don't want the junk others are eating around you. You may find a fresh nut roast with a tomato coulis is just about the best tasting thing imaginable. (This is not as far fetched as it sounds – your taste buds are currently over tuned to sweets and refined carbohydrates. You cannot imagine the sweetness of butternut squash or melon until you have freed yourself from your current habits).

6) *I really want that chocolate bar, muffin, tub of ice cream.*

Of course you do. You are physically craving it. You are addicted to it so you want it as badly as a smoker wants a cigarette or an alcoholic wants a drink. You would do anything to get it, which is precisely why you must not have it. You must not give in. You need to break the addiction, otherwise you will continue to have your life ruled by food and will continue to overeat and be overweight for life. You will also continue to be dopey, bloated, exhausted and everything else that goes with food addiction. All your energy needs to be focused on not giving in to the cravings and ending the addiction.

7) *I'm going to a dinner party tonight – it would be rude not to eat whatever is put in front of me.*

If you are in Phase 1 – what are you doing going to a dinner party? You need to make these five days as easy as possible, not set yourself up to fail.

If you are in Phase 2 you should be fine going for a fat meal option. Just skip the bread and potatoes and fill up on prawn cocktail, casserole, meat, fish, vegetables and any fat/protein that is offered. Hopefully you know your hosts well enough to let them know that you are doing something positive for your weight and your health. If they are good hosts and care about you then they will be understanding and accommodating. A good host does not push dessert on someone trying to lose weight. They do everything that they can to make their guests feel comfortable and relaxed. Hosts are used to coping with vegetarians, genuine food allergies and wheat free diets. If you let your hosts know that you are there to see them, and any carbohydrate free food that they can offer will be a bonus, you will be fine.

In Phase 3 you have a choice – you can still decline the refined carbohydrates, if you choose, but you may choose to accept any whole-meal carbohydrates that are on offer. Or, you could decide to eat what you want, enjoy the freedom for the evening and then get back on track the next day. You are likely to get to a point when eating refined carbohydrates makes you feel so sluggish that you just don't want to do it anymore.

8) *It shouldn't go to waste*

If you are worried about food at home going to waste – why is stuff you might crave there? Stop buying refined carbohydrates. Get rid of all refined carbohydrates at home before you start Phase 1. Your family need to support you – they can benefit from healthier eating too. No one in your family, or any other family for that matter, needs refined carbohydrates so have the **un**refined versions to hand instead.

If you are worried about the children's leftovers try to understand why. Does this come from your own childhood? Are you carrying a subconscious 'rule' that plates must be licked clean? Children, unlike adults, tend to have a natural appetite and they will stop eating as soon as they feel full. If you often get leftovers then reduce the portion sizes served. If it happens just with certain foods then let them decide how much they want of that food (if any). If it happens every now and again just throw the food away or save it for later if it will keep. The food was

223

supposed to be in your child's tummy by now so why should it matter throwing it away? Don't let any daft views on waste ruin your health.

9) *I'm on holiday or I'm in a restaurant – I won't get the chance to eat all of this lovely stuff tomorrow.*

You also won't have a chance to be slim tomorrow unless you start taking control of your eating today. Also – you will actually have a chance to eat all this 'lovely stuff' again. You can come back to the restaurant, or return to the same holiday resort, in the future. Food doesn't ever go away. How often have you eaten something because it was there not because you needed or even wanted it? If there is a box of chocolates, or a celebration cake, being shared out at work don't give in. You can buy and eat an entire box of chocolates or cake on your own tomorrow if you want – I bet you won't want to once the moment has passed. Remember, in Phase 1 and 2, you are trying to get your cravings under control so that you can get back in control of your eating and reach your natural weight. You will be able to eat what you want **almost** when you want in Phase 3. You will be able to sample new foods on holiday. You will be able to indulge in a restaurant. You will be able to have cake and chocolates for celebrations, if this is what you want to do. You will be at your natural weight, your eating will be under control and you will enjoy these indulgences so much more because you will not feel guilty or loathe yourself for having them.

10) *Why not?*

Why not indeed? This is your life. The choice is yours. So often we look for a magic wand or for someone else to make the decisions for us in life. The decision to overeat or to get your eating in control is entirely within your hands. It is up to you. If you really want that chocolate brownie more than you want to be slim then eat it. It really is up to you. However, just stop for one moment before you do eat it and ask yourself why you want it so badly. You are an addict remember. You are not just choosing that chocolate brownie, therefore, you are choosing a way of life. You are choosing to continue to be a food addict, to continue your cravings and to continue to overeat. If you really do want to get to the point where food doesn't rule your life then you have to start by saying no to it now. The longer you say yes, the longer you will be addicted and the harder this will be to overcome when you eventually do tackle it (and you will have to for the sake of your health sooner or later). Why prolong the inevitable any longer? Say no to the craving now and say yes to a craving free future.

KEY POINTS FROM CHAPTER 23

- **It's up to you!**
- No one else is going to make you stop overeating. You have to do it. This book will help you understand the physical reasons for food addiction and cravings. This section, on the psychological aspects of overeating, can help you understand your emotional reasons for eating. But, at the end of the day, you are the one who has to use all of this and make it happen.
- You must believe that you can do this because you absolutely can.
- Finally, you must do it now. Candida, Food Intolerance and Hypoglycaemia do not get better. They do not stay at a steady state. Unless treated they get worse. You have to deal with this some time and the longer you leave it the worse it will be, so sort it now!

PART 7

OTHER RELATED ISSUES

24

"I'M PAT AND I'M AN ALCOHOLIC"

How Candida, Food Intolerance and
Hypoglycaemia explain alcoholism

If you are concerned that you may be an alcoholic as well as a food addict, this chapter could change your life. The principles in this book have huge relevance for people suffering from alcoholism. Alcoholics are not greedy or weak willed. They are suffering an addiction just like smokers, drug addicts and food addicts.

Addiction to alcohol has the same four main characteristics as addiction to any other substance:
1) An uncontrollable craving for alcohol.
2) Increasing tolerance so that more alcohol is needed in order to produce the same effects.
3) Physical or psychological dependence – alcohol starts to give a feeling of well-being (euphoria in the extreme) when you first consume it and then, in the latter stages of the addiction, alcohol is needed to avoid unpleasant withdrawal feelings.
4) Adverse effects on the consumer.

There are further **behavioural** characteristics that define alcoholism which are well documented...
- alcoholics drink alone,
- alcoholics drink early in the day,
- alcoholics drink to feel different – not just because they enjoy the drink,
- alcoholics won't attend certain functions, or do certain things, without having a drink first and so on. The behavioural characteristics are of less concern to us than the physical characteristics, as this book is much more about the physical reasons for addiction than the psychological ones.
Regarding the physical addiction, the critical thing to note about alcoholism is that **an alcoholic is addicted to the ingredients in alcohol and not just the alcohol itself**. A food addict with an addiction to wheat craves biscuits, cakes, pasta, bread and so on. However they

are craving the wheat in biscuits, cakes, pasta and bread and not necessarily the other ingredients. If a wheat addict gives up pasta (which is clearly wheat and not much else) but continues to eat biscuits, they will continue to feed their addiction to wheat and will continue to crave wheat. I suggest that the alcoholic who craves alcohol is actually craving the ingredients in alcohol and not just the general category of alcohol itself. This is hugely significant.

The alcoholic is advised to go 'cold turkey' and to cut out all alcohol, but what if it is the **ingredients** in alcohol that are being craved as part of Candida, Food Intolerance or Hypoglycaemia? In this situation the alcoholic may stop drinking alcohol but they may still be consuming the ingredients that they are addicted to on a daily, if not almost hourly, basis.

To understand how likely this is, let us look at the key ingredients in alcohol:

Wine & champagne are primarily made from grapes which end up in a highly concentrated form (i.e. refined fruit).

Beer is a fermented, hop flavoured, malt sugared liquid whose chief ingredients are water, malt, hops & yeast. (Malting is a process of bringing grain to its highest point of possible soluble starch content. This forms 'maltose'– a sugar – which is then metabolised into alcohol by the yeast).

Lager (from the German word lagern which means to store) is just beer kept in a cold dark place for thirty days or more.

Whisky & Gin are grain based (barley, oats and wheat) and generally contain sugar in addition.

Vodka used to be distilled from potatoes but is more typically grain based today.

Rum has sugar cane as its key ingredient. (As a sweet addict do you find yourself loving rum & coke?)

Hence the key ingredients in alcohol are sugar, yeast, grains and concentrated fruit sugar. These are some of the most common causes of Candida, Food Intolerance and Hypoglycaemia. Let us now look at each of these in turn:

Candida – it is extremely likely that alcoholics will be suffering from Candida having consumed yeast and sugar in such quantities over a period of time.

Food Intolerance – it is most likely that Food Intolerance to sugar, yeast and grains has built up over time during the period of high alcohol consumption.

Hypoglycaemia – the impact of alcohol being a stimulant, along with the impact that alcohol has on blood glucose hormones, means that Hypoglycaemia is likely to also be playing a part.

If someone wants to have a real chance of overcoming addiction to alcohol, therefore, they need to overcome the Candida, Food Intolerance and Hypoglycaemia that are almost certainly accompanying the alcoholism.

If alcoholics avoid all yeast, sugar, grapes and grains during the first few days of giving up alcohol they will find that they recover from cravings far sooner than if they continue to consume the **ingredients** of alcohol but just not alcohol itself. Alcoholics need to make sure that they overcome the Candida, Food Intolerance and Hypoglycaemia related to the ingredients in alcohol before adding these ingredients back into their diets.

The other enormous implication of this approach is that alcoholics may not need to give up alcohol for ever. If they free themselves of their addiction to the ingredients in alcohol they may be able to drink alcohol again in the future provided that they don't drink too much or too often. If they return to drinking alcohol in significant quantities every day they will have problems again very quickly. However, if they don't drink too much or too often they may be able to return to the social drinking that they were once able to enjoy before the addiction took hold.

KEY POINTS FROM CHAPTER 24
- Alcoholics, drug addicts and food addicts have very similar problems.
- The ingredients in alcoholic drinks are invariably the ones that cause Candida, Food Intolerance and Hypoglycaemia.
- If an alcoholic gives up their favourite drink, but continues to consume the ingredients in that drink in every day foods, they will continue to have huge cravings for alcohol. Alcoholics need to give up the ingredients that they are intolerant to at the same time that they give up alcohol to free themselves from cravings.

25

"ANIMALS ARE MY FRIENDS AND I DON'T EAT MY FRIENDS"

Can you follow this plan and still be vegetarian?

I have been a vegetarian for over ten years – much to the dismay of every nutritionist I have worked with. They have all asked if I would consider eating fish as they said that this would be good for my health. I am a vegetarian because I love animals and can't bear the thought of eating them but my most important personal value is health so I do have a dilemma here.

If you are suffering from Candida it will be very difficult for you to overcome this condition whilst being a vegetarian. It will be close to impossible as a vegan. As the most basic anti-Candida eating plan is meat/fish, eggs, salad, vegetables and Natural Live Yoghurt, if you do not eat any animal foods you will not be able to launch a strong dietary onslaught against Candida. Vegans would have to live on vegetables to adhere to the strict anti-Candida eating plan and this would not be healthy, or give them anywhere near enough energy.

Vegetarians will struggle on Phase 1 but Phase 2 actually lends itself very well to vegetarianism. In Phase 1, vegetarians will need to eat a lot of eggs and Natural Live Yoghurt to ensure that they get enough to eat, along with unlimited salad, vegetables and a limited quantity of brown rice. In Phase 2, vegetarians can continue to eat eggs – but will probably want to cut back on the quantities – and they can then have brown rice vegetarian dishes or whole-wheat pasta with vegetable sauces or baked potatoes and low fat filling. They can eat all pulses and dairy products. The carbohydrate meals in Phase 2 are always vegetarian as they omit animal fat.

If you are a fish eater, you will be fine with all phases of the eating plans. In Phase 1 you can have Kedgeree (fish and brown rice) for breakfast, fish and vegetables for lunch and brown rice and vegetables for dinner. You can snack on tins of tuna if you get hungry.

Meat eaters are also fine at every phase of the programme – they have the most choice of all. However, they may find the carbohydrate/vegetable meals a bit alien. If this is the case, stick with meat, fish, vegetables and salad. Your weight loss will be even quicker if you do as you will be minimising the impact on the release of insulin into your body.

The bottom line, therefore, is that you can follow this eating plan and be a vegetarian. However, if you have a significant problem with Candida you should seriously consider eating fish for a period of time just to get your Candida back under control. You can always go back to being a vegetarian as soon as your immune system has recovered and the Candida is back in balance. If you really cannot face the thought of eating fish try Phase 1 with lots of eggs, salad, vegetables, Natural Live Yoghurt and a higher allocation of brown rice. Hopefully this will kill off the Candida and give you enough to eat in the process.

KEY POINTS FROM CHAPTER 25
- Vegetarians will struggle with Phase 1 of the eating plan and vegans even more so.
- However, you can still be a vegetarian and follow this plan as I have done for years.
- If Candida is a real problem for you, you may like to take nutritional advice and see if your conscience will allow you to eat fish just until such time as your own health is back under control.

26

SO CAN YOU BIN THE GYM MEMBERSHIP?

Where does exercise fit in with all of this?

Let us go back to the calorie theory to answer this question. There are approximately 250 calories in an average confectionery bar. To 'burn off' those calories, a 150lb person would need to do the following:
- Run for 24 minutes,
- Cycle for 37 minutes,
- Weight train for 53 minutes,
- Walk for 42 minutes,
- Aerobics for 33-38 minutes,
- Swim for 29 minutes.

The general guidelines are that we use up the following calories per pound of body weight per hour:
- Running uses up 4.2 calories per pound of body weight per hour,
- Cycling (at 10 miles per hour) uses up 2.7,
- Weight training uses up 1.9,
- Walking (at 2.4 miles per hour) uses up 2.4,
- Aerobics uses up 2.6-3,
- Swimming (slow freestyle) uses up 3.5.

I love swimming, but, if I didn't, I would rather forego the confectionery bar than feel I had to swim for half an hour afterwards to burn it off!

If you remember, the calorie theory tells you to drive from one end of the country to the other but without putting enough petrol in your car. The exercise part of the calorie theory tells you to increase your level of activity so that your car needs even more petrol! The calorie theory tells you to exercise because it wants you to eat less than your body needs and it wants you to increase the amount your body needs so that this deficit increases even further. i.e. it wants you to be hungry and it wants you to exercise more so that you are even hungrier! It is not surprising that this makes you crave food.

Because you don't believe the calorie theory you don't need to exercise with this eating plan. You don't count calories. You know that counting calories doesn't work and, worse still, makes you fat. You don't **need** to exercise because you are not trying to increase your need for food or increase the gap between the calories you eat and the calories you need. You are focusing on **what** you eat, not **how much,** so you don't need to exercise to make this eating plan work.

However, forget whether or not you need to exercise for your weight and exercise because it is a great thing to do. There are so many benefits of exercise that you should find something you enjoy and do it regularly. Whether it is swimming, yoga, walking or cycling, or any one of the many team sports around, there are huge benefits to be reaped from being active:

- You will have more energy and will be able to live life to the full.
- You will be fitter and more able to do everyday activities with ease.
- Your body will be more toned and will look slimmer whatever size you are.
- You will ease stress levels and find it easier to relax.
- You will develop and maintain the three key aspects of fitness – strength, stamina and suppleness.
- You will have fun and opportunities to socialise depending on the type of exercise that you choose.
- You may have an animal that will greatly enjoy you spending more time exercising with them. Even cats love their owners being outside with them exploring their territory.
- There is a complete aura of vitality around people who are fit and active, whatever their size.

One of the best things about exercise, apart from the fact that it makes you feel good, is that it builds muscle and stimulates your metabolism so your general body engine works better on the fuel that it is given. Think of it as like giving your car a regular service. So, exercise for any of the above reasons but not because you want to use up calories.

As a final point – remember that this book is about insulin and how this is the fattening hormone. Because exercise has little impact on insulin this is another reason why exercise isn't needed for this eating plan to work. In fact the opposite is true. Exercise actually lowers your blood glucose level so watch out for cravings afterwards. Have a piece of fruit handy and lots of water to drink so that you can get your fluid and blood glucose level naturally back in balance.

KEY POINTS FROM CHAPTER 26

- Don't exercise because you want to increase your need for calories. Calorie counting doesn't work and worse still it makes you fat!
- Exercise because it is a wonderful thing to do for your body, stress levels and overall well-being.

PART 8

QUESTIONS & ANSWERS

80 FREQUENTLY ASKED QUESTIONS
WITH STRAIGHT TALKING ANSWERS

PART 8

80 FREQUENTLY ASKED QUESTIONS...

The bottom line

Q1) Why do you overeat? – When all you want is to be slim.

A) Because you have cravings that are so strong you might as well be a heroin addict trying to give up heroin or a smoker trying to give up cigarettes. You are not weak willed or greedy. You are fighting a force on an hourly basis that would beat the strongest of wills.

You have these cravings because of one thing that you are doing and because of one, or all, of three conditions that you may have:

- The one thing that you are doing is calorie counting. As soon as you try to eat less fuel than your body needs, you will crave food as this is your body's way of making you eat to give it the fuel that it needs.

- The conditions that you may have, which are causing your cravings, are Candida, Food Intolerance and Hypoglycaemia. Candida drives you to crave sugary, yeasty and vinegary foods. Food Intolerance drives you to crave anything to which you are intolerant – this can literally be any food or drink from eggs to alcohol. Hypoglycaemia drives you to crave refined carbohydrates, as your blood glucose level rises and falls on an hourly basis. You need to eliminate refined carbohydrates and any foods to which you are intolerant, to overcome the cravings. Once the cravings subside you will then have the chance to reach a healthy weight and stay there long term.

Q2) Why have I failed so many times before?

A) Because of the cravings – you know how strong they have been. They have been incredible forces to get in the way of the thing that you most want – to be slim. Remember the trips to the all night grocery store or the petrol/gas station. Remember driving out of your way to get a particular food or drink. You have been an addict, who has been told to eat everything in moderation – about as sensible as telling an alcoholic to have one drink and no more.

Q3) Why will I succeed this time?

A) Because you now have the power of knowledge. You know why you have failed before – because of the cravings. You know what you have been craving and why. You know that the cravings have come from calorie counting, Candida, Food Intolerance and Hypoglycaemia. You know that you have to eliminate the offending foods from your diet to make the cravings disappear.

Q4) How much weight will I lose?

A) This will be different for every person. Gender plays a part – men tend to lose more weight on diets than women. The more you have to lose the more you will lose. The more conditions you have been suffering from, the more you will lose. Food Intolerance and Candida in particular are known to play havoc with water retention so, after just five days on the kick-start eating plan, you could lose half a stone or even more. The key thing is that you will tend towards your natural weight quickly and safely. You will eat healthy whole foods that nourish you and you will not be hungry. Some of my case studies have had stones to lose and they have lost stones and kept them off. The record weight loss to date has been 14lb on phase 1! This has been achieved on several occasions.

Q5) How is this eating plan different from others?

A) It meets all the criteria for a successful eating plan:
- It works.
- It is practical.
- It is long term.
- It is healthy.
- It is enjoyable.

You can't live on cakes and chocolate all day long and be the weight you want to be. You are overweight because of food cravings so you have to overcome these. What this eating plan will do is to overcome the cravings so you will no longer think that life is incomplete without sweet things and refined carbohydrates. You will then be able to enjoy the wide variety of healthy foods that you can eat on a long term basis.

This eating plan is also the first to directly understand cravings – why you get them, what causes them, what impact calorie controlled diets have on them and how to get rid of them. It is also the first book to directly link Candida, Food Intolerance and Hypoglycaemia with food cravings and to complete the jigsaw of factors in modern day life which explain why obesity is at epidemic levels.

Q6)   What medical bits do I need to know?

A) Chapter 2 tries to keep the medical bits to the minimum. The key thing to take away from this book is that it is insulin, not calories, which makes you fat. Insulin is a hormone that is released by the pancreas when you eat something that raises your blood glucose level. The pancreas releases insulin to get your blood glucose level back to 'normal'. If it didn't do this you would be diabetic.

Q7)   Why is insulin called the fattening hormone?

A) When we eat carbohydrates, our body decides how much of the energy taken in is needed immediately and how much should be stored for future requirements. As our blood glucose level rises, insulin is released from the pancreas and this insulin converts some of the glucose to glycogen. Glycogen is our energy store room. **If all the glycogen storage areas are full, insulin will convert the excess to fatty tissue. This is why insulin has been called the fattening hormone.**

Cravings

Q8)   Why have I had these cravings?

A) If you have been calorie counting you have probably just been hungry. Because of your body's incredible survival instinct, it has been trying to get you to eat (anything) just to maintain the fuel levels that it needs to survive. The activity of calorie counting alone has led to cravings.

On top of this, calorie counting has depleted your nutrients and weakened your immune system. This, with or without other factors such as taking the birth control pill, or antibiotics or having had extreme stress, can lead to any, or all, of Candida, Food Intolerance and Hypoglycaemia. You only need one of these conditions and you will have cravings as strong as any faced by a drug addict.

Q9)   Will they go away?

A) Yes! Everything is within your power. First you need to stop calorie counting. This may require a change in your mind set but you have nothing to lose and everything to gain. Then all of the conditions – Candida, Food Intolerance and Hypoglycaemia – can be controlled in the short and long term. The other thing to remember is, if you don't start to control these conditions they will only get worse. So the sooner you tackle this, the better. Look at the tips for positive thinking in Part 9 and be determined to crack this. One of the best tips for motivation is that unless you plan to live your entire life overweight and exhausted you are going to have to crack this some time. Why not start now?

Q10) When will they go away?

A) The good news is that you can significantly reduce food cravings quite quickly. In just five days on a new eating plan you can do the following:
- You can stop counting calories and thereby stop your body demanding fuel.
- You can have a major impact on the Candida overgrowth in your body and dramatically reduce the cravings for yeasty, vinegary and sugary foods.
- You can eliminate the foods to which you are intolerant and clear any traces of these from your system, leading to a dramatic reduction in cravings.
- You can stabilise your blood glucose level in fewer than five days – even a day's healthy eating can start the stabilisation of your blood glucose level.

The first five days will be tough but you really can achieve a dramatic reduction in cravings in this short time period. Without the cravings trying to ruin your good intentions your will power is free to take you to the success you have always dreamed of.

Q11) How do I stop 'good' days and 'bad' days?

A) By this you mean bingeing and starving. The key is to stop either one of 'good' days or 'bad' days as one leads directly to the other. You only try to have a 'good' day to lose the weight you gain after a 'bad' day. And you only have bad days when you are so hungry and deprived after a day of calorie restriction. It doesn't matter which one you vow to stop – starve days or binge days – one leads to the other so stopping one stops the other.

Q12) How do I stop being a food addict?

A) By stopping the food cravings. This in turn is done by stopping calorie counting and by making sure that any problems you have with Candida, Food Intolerance and/or Hypoglycaemia are addressed. You must stop eating the foods that you crave – easier said than done I hear you say and you are right – but this is the only way to stop the food cravings. Now that you understand what you crave and why, you have the power to overcome food addiction.

What I thought I knew

Q13) Why does everyone tell me to count calories?

A) Why do people smoke when it is a well known fact that smoking kills one in two people who use the product, over time, exactly as it is intended to be used by the manufacturers? I struggle to answer this one as it just doesn't make sense. I think just as it has taken us years to realise that smoking is probably the worst thing we can do for our health, so it will take us years to get rid of the calorie myth.

The calorie myth was first proposed in 1930 and it has received little challenge since. Even the proposers of the theory were alarmed at how literally their research was adopted and applied back in the 1930's. They followed up their initial research with words of caution but the bandwagon was already rolling by this time. The calorie theory has been proven not to work in practice as the fewer calories we have been eating as nations, the fatter we have got. One of the most important things to take out of this book is a changed way of thinking. If you read this book and still think counting calories is the answer I have failed and you will continue to fail. You **must** throw out this myth and see how counting calories leads to food cravings, lower metabolism and increased weight rather than reduced weight.

People tell you to count calories because they think that if your body takes in less fuel than it needs you will lose weight. You now know that if you take in less fuel than your body needs the first thing that your body will do is to crave food to get you to eat more. The next thing that your body will do is to become weaker, less healthy and less able to resist problems such as Candida, Food Intolerance and Hypoglycaemia and then your cravings will be amplified further still. You also know that if you count calories you will simply slow down your metabolism making weight loss harder still.

Q14) Why can't I still count calories?

A) Because if you continue to count calories you will continue to try to restrict them. If you start to find yourself eating 2000 calories a day, or more, you will consciously, or subconsciously, try to cut back. The hardest thing that you will do, in following the eating advice in this book, is to give up your 'prop' of counting calories. Your key goal now is to stop cravings, not to count calories. If you try to eat fewer calories than your body needs you will crave food and it is the food cravings that are making you overweight. After reading this book, if you still think calories make you fat then eat no carbohydrate whatsoever for a few days. Eat as much fat/protein as you can manage and see how much weight you lose. I expect it will be pounds. Then ask yourself how you can eat so many calories and still lose weight – because calories are fuel for your body not bad things that make you fat.

Q15) Won't I put on weight if I don't count calories?

A)No! You will put on weight if you continue to crave food like an addict and give into those cravings. Your number one objective now has to be to stop cravings, not to count calories. Put all your effort into stopping the cravings by getting your Candida, Food Intolerance and Hypoglycaemia under control and by not counting calories, which makes you crave anything. You are going to stop eating the foods that have been making you fat so you will not put on weight. You will be nourishing your body and giving it what it needs, which is going to help it find its natural and healthy weight.

Q16) Should I count carbohydrates…?

A) No! Don't count anything – just put all that energy that used to be spent counting calories into craving control. Your number one goal now is to stop cravings. Do that and everything else will follow.

Q17) …or fat units?

A) No! See above answer.

Q18) I have been told if I stop eating certain things I will crave them more – many diets advise me to have a little bit of what I fancy – why is this book saying to avoid certain foods?

A) How crazy is this? Is the heroin addict told to have just a bit of heroin but not too much? Is the alcoholic told to have just one drink but not the whole bottle? The food addict would be a lot better off if they could go cold turkey on food just as the drug addict, alcoholic and smoker can. We can't stop eating but we can stop eating certain foods – the ones causing us problems. Sugar does nothing positive for our health whatsoever so we will lose nothing by giving it up. Similarly there are **un**refined alternatives for all refined carbohydrates and we will always be better off nutritionally by eating the whole-meal alternatives to refined food.

Having read this book you should know that you are craving food because of one, or all, of calorie counting, Candida, Food Intolerance or Hypoglycaemia. Unless you stop eating the foods that are causing these conditions and food cravings, your cravings will get steadily worse not better. Remember that the 'devil' in your head is telling you to eat the food(s) to which you are addicted so this voice will jump on any magazine article that says that you can eat a bit of what you fancy. This is what you want to believe.

Finally, another response to this question is that a little bit of what you fancy is OK when you are at your natural weight and when you are free from Candida, Food Intolerance and Hypoglycaemia and your immune system is able to cope with refined carbohydrates. Until then, a little bit of what you fancy will lead to a lot of what you fancy and it will keep you where you are now.

Carbohydrates

Q19) Why are refined carbohydrates the baddies?

A) Just to get this totally clear – carbohydrates are not the baddies. **Refined** carbohydrates are the baddies. Fruit, whole-meal grains and vegetables are all carbohydrates but they are not refined so they have goodness and nutrients within them. Fats have always been around and they are an essential part of our diet. Cave people lived on fruits, berries and animal products and we have no reason to believe that they suffered obesity, Candida, Food Intolerance or Hypoglycaemia.

It is since we have introduced manufactured foods to our diet that we have had problems. Grains have been a relatively recent addition to our diets (in the past couple of hundred years) and these are, therefore, less familiar to our bodies than the foods our ancestors lived on. Products like sugar and food additives and preservatives, and the other many things we ingest today, are even worse. There is a scale of foods, therefore, from the most natural foods like fruits, berries and animal products that we have eaten for centuries and at the other end of the scale, processed foods that are amongst the most recent additions to our diets and are, therefore, quite alien to our bodies.

Refined carbohydrates are the baddies for the following reasons:
- They are low in nutrients,
- They are alien to our bodies and most importantly to our pancreas,
- They stimulate the production of insulin, which is the fattening hormone,

- They contribute to Candida, Food Intolerance and Hypoglycaemia and these in turn can lead to food cravings and weight gain,
- If we consume refined carbohydrates we will either be overeating other foods to get the nutrients that we need, or we will be deficient in some nutrients.

Q20) How do I know what is a refined food and what isn't?

A) The simple answer is that if a food is as it would be found in its natural form it is OK. If a food has been altered in some way from its natural form it is not OK. Here are some examples:
- Brown rice and brown, whole-wheat, pasta are OK; white rice and white pasta have been altered further by food processing so they are **not** OK.
- Brown, whole-wheat, flour is OK; white flour has been further processed and is **not** OK.
- Bread made from whole-wheat flour, with no sugar or any of its derivatives, is OK; white bread, or any bread with added refined ingredients, is **not** OK.
- Pure, fresh meat and fish are OK; processed and packaged meat and fish is **not** OK.
- Fruit, as it is found on trees, is fine; fruit juice or dried fruit isn't because this is not how it is found in its natural form. (Cartons of fruit juice do not grow on trees!)

Q21) What about potatoes – friend or foe?

A) Potatoes have had a mixed reaction in diet books. The book *"Potatoes not Prozac"*, by Kathleen DesMaisons, shows how the natural serotonin in potatoes makes us feel good. Michel Montignac points to the high glycaemic index of potatoes and advises us not to go near them. The advice in this book is that the whole potato is OK as it is **un**refined (i.e. a jacket potato in its skin) but the refined versions of potatoes are not – chips, crisps etc. Baked jacket potatoes are a useful food for office workers as invariably people have a baked potato bar near work and can, therefore, get a practical hot meal for lunch. Also, a lot of offices have microwaves and you can bring in partially baked potatoes to heat up at lunchtime. Remember the potato is a carbohydrate meal, however, so don't mix it with fat – no butter, therefore, no cheese. You can have low fat cottage cheese, salad, ratatouille or vegetables – you get the idea.

Q22) Pasta vs rice?

A) Rice, for Europeans and Americans, is rarely a food to which we are intolerant as we don't eat it often enough to become intolerant to it. Pasta, however, is often a food to which we are intolerant as it is from the wheat family which we tend to eat at every meal – breakfast cereal, toast, sandwiches, bread, pizza, beer and so on. It is quite likely, therefore, that you will need to avoid wheat in Phase 2, if these are the foods that you crave. You can try some whole-wheat pasta as part of Phase 2 but if you find it causes your lethargy or cravings to return, you will know you have identified a problem food. You will probably be safe with rice however. You can have some brown rice with Phase 1 and try to make rice, rather than pasta, your staple carbohydrate during Phase 2. Brown rice is so delicious and versatile as a grain. You can make paella, Chinese vegetable dishes, Mexican chilli style dishes, vegetable curries and so on. Remember rice is a carbohydrate meal so you must eat this with vegetables and not fat. You can use some vegetable fat in cooking – e.g. stir-fry vegetables in olive oil – but no other fat.

Q23) Why is sugar the number one baddie?

A) Because it does nothing positive for our bodies and it does a lot that is negative instead. It gives us no vitamins or minerals of any significance and it depletes our stock of vitamins and minerals in its digestion. It upsets blood glucose balance, stimulates insulin production and gives us nothing back in return. Sugar is 'empty calories' so we still need to eat more calories to get the nutrients that we need. It also tastes so sweet that it disturbs our taste buds for naturally sweets foods like fruit and vegetables. It is the only substance that we eat or drink that gives us virtually no nutrients whatsoever.

Q24) What is sugar in? wheat? milk?

A) Please see Chapter 17 which has full details of where all kinds of substances can be found in everyday foods.

Fats

Q25) Why is fat OK to eat?

A) We need fat for all the cells in our bodies. Without the fat and fatty acids that our bodies need we will suffer all kinds of health complaints from minor ones, such as dry skin, to major ones such as strokes or growth retardation. Fat has got its bad reputation from the calorie myth in that people think if fat has 9 calories per gram and carbohydrate has 4 calories per gram then we are better off eating carbohydrate. We now know that the calorie theory doesn't work, that insulin is the fattening hormone and that fat doesn't stimulate insulin production whereas carbohydrate consumption does. Our ancestors ate most of their food in the form of fat and protein as they lived on animals and animal products. Hence fat has to be a key part of our eating plans. In summary, therefore, we need fat, it doesn't make us fat, we have lived on fat for hundreds of years and it performs several vital functions within our bodies.

Q26) Are there good fats and bad fats?

A)   Yes – the good fats, which we need, are:
- Polyunsaturated fats which lower bad cholesterol and provide the Essential Fatty Acids Omega 3 and Omega 6. These are found in seeds, fish and their oils.
- Monounsaturated fats which lower overall cholesterol. These are found in olive oil and canola oil.
The very bad fats, which we should totally avoid, are:
- Transunsaturated fats which lower good cholesterol, raise bad cholesterol and raise overall cholesterol. These are found in margarine, manufactured fats, shortening and anywhere where you see the description 'hydrogenated' fats.
The not-so-good fats, which we should eat with caution, are:
- Saturated fats which raise bad and total cholesterol, though they have no impact on good cholesterol. These are found in animal foods like meat and dairy products.

The Conditions
Candida – Chapter 9

Q27) What is Candida?

A) Candida is a yeast that exists in all of us which is normally controlled by our immune system and other bacterial flora present in our body. It usually resides in the digestive tract. Candida serves no useful purpose in the body and can, therefore, be viewed as a parasite. In many people this yeast causes no harm and lives within us peacefully. The issue is when Candida multiplies out of control and causes significant impact on our health and well-being.

Q28)　What causes Candida?

A) Or put another way – if yeast can multiply to frightening levels given the right environment – what makes our body the right environment for Candida to multiply? There are five key things that do this:
1) A weakened immune system,
2) Over-consumption of refined carbohydrates,
3) Medication – steroids, antibiotics, birth control pills, hormones,
4) Diabetes,
5) Nutritional deficiency.
Please see Chapter 9 for full details of all of these.

Q29)　How do I know if I have Candida?

A) In general, chronic Candida overgrowth can make a person feel very unwell all over. Here are some of the many symptoms that you may be experiencing if you have Candida overgrowth:

Stomach – constipation; diarrhoea; irritable bowel syndrome; stomach distension; bloating, especially after eating; two sets of clothes needed for pre and post eating; indigestion; gas; heartburn.

Head – headaches; dizziness; earaches; blurred vision; flushed cheeks; feeling of 'sleepwalking'; feeling unreal; feeling 'spaced out'.

Women – Pre-Menstrual Tension (PMT); water retention; irregular menstruation; painful breasts; vaginal discharge or itchiness; thrush; cystitis.

Blood Glucose – hungry between meals; irritable or moody before meals; shaky when hungry; faintness when food is not eaten; irregular pulse before and after eating; headaches late morning; waking in the early hours and not being able to get back to sleep; abnormal cravings for sweet foods, bread, alcohol or caffeine; eating sweets increases hunger; excessive appetite; instant sugar 'high' followed by fatigue; chilly feeling after eating.

Mental – anxiety; depression; irritability; lethargy; memory problems; loss of concentration; moodiness; nightmares; mental 'sluggishness'; "*get up and go*" has got up and gone.

Other – athletes foot; dandruff or other fungal infections; Food Intolerance; dramatic fluctuations in weight from one day to the next; poor circulation; hands and feet sensitive to cold; exhaustion; feeling of being unable to cope; constant fatigue; muscle aches; susceptibility to infection; gasping for breath; sighing often – 'hunger for air'; tightness in chest; chest aches; cramps; yawning easily; insomnia; excessive thirst; easy weight gain; coated tongue; dry skin; hair loss; symptoms worse after consuming yeast or sugary foods; symptoms worse on damp, humid or rainy days.

Q30) How does Candida cause food cravings?

A) Candida is a living organism and every living thing has a natural self-preservation mechanism – we all fight to survive. The yeast living inside us is no exception. The Candida needs refined carbohydrates to feed it, it thrives on a weak immune system, it hates garlic and nutrients as they attack it and kill it off. You are having a constant battle with your body, therefore. You are trying to feel well but the Candida is trying to survive. The things needed for your well-being and the Candida's well-being are opposite.

When Candida really takes hold you will crave the foods that feed the yeast to ensure it grows and flourishes – all sugary foods, refined carbohydrates, concentrated fruit sugar, yeast and yeast derivatives and vinegary/pickled foods. There is evidence to suggest that yeast itself does not feed the yeast but the consumption of bread and other foods containing yeast generally maintains the environment that the yeast needs to thrive in your body.

Q31) How can you treat Candida?

A) There are three key pieces of advice for people suffering from Candida:
1) Starve the Candida overgrowth with diet,
2) Attack the Candida overgrowth with supplements that kill the yeast,
3) Treat the causes so that it doesn't come back.

Q32) How can I stop Candida coming back?

A) By remembering the key causes of Candida and ensuring that you do not re-create the environment for yeast overgrowth in your body. This means:
1) Keeping you and your immune system healthy,
2) Not consuming too many carbohydrates, especially refined ones,
3) Avoiding hormones and antibiotics wherever possible,
4) Managing your blood glucose level, whether diabetic or not, and
5) Getting all the vitamins and minerals that you need.

Q33) Why is fruit restricted in the eating plans for Candida?

A) The advice on Candida to date has been to restrict fruit totally for a few weeks and quite significantly for some time thereafter. This advice is given because fruit is a carbohydrate and any carbohydrate, especially sweet fruits, can feed the yeast. Starving the yeast of the foods it needs to survive means avoiding all sugars, including fruit sugar, for a period of time.

The advice varies in terms of the period for which fruit sugar should be avoided. Some practitioners advise weeks, if not months, without fruit. This undoubtedly will help with Candida, but there are more factors to consider in relation to your overall well-being. Fruit is so rich in fibre, vitamins and minerals that it is too good a food to avoid for a long period of time. In this book we avoid fruit just for the 5 day kick-start eating plan to have a quick and significant impact on Candida. If you are not that keen on fruit, then you can continue to avoid it for as long as Candida causes you a problem. However, if you like fruit, it is more important for your eating plan to be enjoyable, practical and something you can stick to. Many people, women in particular, would simply not start an eating plan that advised them to avoid fruit for weeks.

Health is an all over concept and if someone is happy and enjoying their food, this is almost as valuable as forcing someone to eat 'the perfect eating plan' whatever that may be. You need to become your own health monitor and balance enjoyment of healthy foods with the knowledge and awareness of foods that cause you problems. If fruit does you more harm than good then restrict it, if not, enjoy it.

Q34) How long should the 'die-off' last (with Candida?)

A) This very much depends on how severe your Candida problem has become. If you have read this book in good time and are tackling the problem early, you may find the first five days uncomfortable but not bad enough to make you feel very unwell. If you have been overeating and craving food for years and have always wondered why, and you now realise that Candida is one of your problems, you could be in for quite a rough time. You could experience die-off for many days or even a few weeks, so be prepared to launch a war on this unwelcome invader.

Try to view 'die-off' as a positive thing – the worse you feel, the more harm you are doing to the yeast and the more you are killing it off. Use the pain of the 'die-off' to strengthen your resolve to rid your body of this hideous invader and to never let it return. See 'die-off' as proof that Candida has been a problem for you and look forward to the time when the yeast and cravings will be back under control and your overeating and excess weight will disappear.

Q35) Is there a medical test for Candida?

A) Some nutritionists do offer stool tests which can detect levels of Candida in the matter excreted by the body. Unless you have a huge desire to send a 'number two' off in a medical container I would advise sticking to the questionnaire in Chapter 9 as this will give you a very good idea of whether or not Candida is an issue for you. There are some Candida support organisations that offer information on blood and saliva tests that are available. Two that you can contact are www.candida-society.org.uk. and www.candidasupport.org. I have also heard of a Do-It-Yourself test for Candida. The test involves spitting into a clear glass of water first thing in the morning and seeing what happens within the next half an hour. If there are 'strings' coming down from your saliva or if the water turns cloudy or if your saliva sinks to the bottom of the glass this has been shown to be a good indication that you have an overgrowth of Candida.

Q36) Will I have Candida for ever?

A) Yes and No. You will always have Candida in your body as it lives within all of us. However, you can get this parasite back in control and stop the huge impact it is having on your health and well-being. You can launch the three pronged attack in Q31 and you can get Candida back in control in your body. The best way to keep Candida at bay is to keep your immune system strong and healthy by eating well, taking a vitamin & mineral tablet daily, doing some exercise regularly that you enjoy and getting balance in your work and play.

Q37) When can I re-introduce more foods?

A) As soon as you know that Candida is not a problem for you (redo the questionnaire in Chapter 9 and see if the many symptoms have subsided), you can re-introduce more foods cautiously to make sure that you keep the Candida under control. Try introducing foods one at a time so that, if the symptoms do return, you will know what has caused this to happen. Try adding baked potatoes to start with. Then add more whole grains, such as whole-wheat pasta if you are OK with wheat. Add in more fruits keeping a close check on how many you can add back in before the symptoms return. If they don't return, this is an excellent sign that your immune system is doing well having been nourished with healthy food.

Q38) What is Food Intolerance?

A) Food Intolerance means, quite literally, not being able to tolerate a particular food or foods. By intolerance we mean an adverse reaction – not an extreme life threatening reaction as with food allergy – but any adverse reaction which causes the person discomfort. Adverse reactions can include anything from gastrointestinal disorders to headaches and reactions which affect the mental state of the person who has consumed the food.

The most common features of Food Intolerance are:

What – Food Intolerance develops with repeated overexposure to a particular food. The key words here are 'repeated' and 'overexposure'. It is most usual for people to become intolerant to foods that they eat a lot of and on a regular basis.

When – Food Intolerance is not fixed as with food allergy and it can vary over time. People can find themselves susceptible to certain foods at different stages of their lives for example. Someone suffering stress can develop an intolerance to a food that they are consuming a lot of at the time and then be able to eat the food again in moderation at other times in their life. The other interesting aspect of Food Intolerance, related to time, is that the adverse reaction is not immediate as with food allergy. For example a person can eat a food to which they are intolerant and develop symptoms over the next twenty-four to forty-eight hours.

How – The offending food produces a state of well-being ranging from a slight mood change to an almost manic state of euphoria. This is when the addictive aspect of Food Intolerance takes hold. Gradually more and more of the offending food is needed to produce the state of well-being provided previously by a normal portion of the food. At this stage necessity has replaced desire.

Q39) What causes Food Intolerance?

A) The clue is in the text above – 'repeated' and 'overexposure'. Anything we eat often and in large quantities we can become intolerant to. It is very rare to be intolerant to something we eat little of and rarely.

There are other things that happen to make us more susceptible to Food Intolerance – illness and medication can lead to a weakened immune system that will make us more susceptible to Food Intolerance and then this in turn weakens our immune system further (we are into the vicious circle at this stage).

Counting calories can also lead to Food Intolerance for a couple of reasons:

- We can weaken our immune system by taking in less fuel than we need.
- We tend to eat a restricted variety of foods when we count calories – we tend to eat more fruit, salad and other low calories foods and cut out steak, full fat dairy products and other higher calorie foods. As we restrict the variety of foods that we eat, sticking to our favourites that fill us up as much as possible for as few calories as possible, we are starting down the slippery slope towards Food Intolerance.

Q40) How do I know if I have Food Intolerance?

A) As with Candida, the range of symptoms related to Food Intolerance are many and varied. There are also remarkable overlaps, which is why so often people with extreme cravings and weight problems are suffering from both conditions. The complaints include:

Stomach – constipation; diarrhoea; irritable bowel syndrome; stomach distension; bloating, especially after eating; two sets of clothes needed for pre and post eating; indigestion; gas; heartburn.

Head – headaches; dizziness; flushed cheeks; feeling of 'sleepwalking'; feeling unreal; feeling 'spaced out'.

Women – PMT; water retention; irregular menstruation.

Blood Glucose – hungry between meals; irritable or moody before meals; shaky when hungry; faintness when food is not eaten; irregular pulse before and after eating; headaches late morning; waking in the early hours and not being able to get back to sleep; abnormal cravings for sweets or caffeine; eating sweets increases hunger; excessive appetite; instant sugar 'high' followed by fatigue; chilly feeling after eating.

Mental – anxiety; depression; irritability; lethargy; memory problems; loss of concentration; moodiness; nightmares; mental 'sluggishness'; "*get up and go*" has got up and gone.

Other – Dramatic fluctuations in weight from one day to the next; exhaustion; feeling of being unable to cope; constant fatigue; muscle aches; susceptibility to infection; gasping for breath; sighing often – 'hunger for air'; chest aches; cramps; excessive thirst; easy weight gain; coated tongue; dry skin; itchiness/rashes.

Q41) How does Food Intolerance cause food cravings?

A) The real irony is that the foods to which you are intolerant are the foods that you crave. Just as the drug addict or smoker craves their fix so you crave the substance that is causing you harm. It starts off with a particular food or drink that you consume on regular occasions. Any substance that you eat daily can start to cause problems and those you eat several times a day are the chief suspects. It takes three to four days for a substance to pass through our bodies, so we can overload our bodies if we eat a substance daily or even more often.

Our bodies then literally become 'intolerant' to the food – i.e. they can't cope with any more of it. You would think that we would shun the food if we had become intolerant to it but in fact the addiction that goes with Food Intolerance actually means that the opposite happens. If we remember back to the definition of addiction we go through these characteristics with Food Intolerance:

- We start with an uncontrollable **craving**,
- We then need more and more of the offending substance in order to get the same 'high' i.e. more **cravings**,
- We develop physical and/or psychological dependence, more **cravings** still!
- We suffer the adverse effects.

Q42) How can you treat Food Intolerance?

A) Step 1, identify the foods to which you are intolerant (by seeing a nutritionist or by keeping a food diary yourself) and Step 2, stop eating them.

Food Intolerance is much easier to spot than you might think. The chances are that the food(s) you crave is/are the one(s) to which you are intolerant. Given that Food Intolerance is caused by **repeated overexposure** to a particular food or food family, the foods that you consume on a regular basis are the ones that you should suspect. Stop eating these for at least five days and then test the food you suspect completely on its own (e.g. 100% shredded wheat to test wheat). If you have a reaction to this food you can be confident that this was one of your problem foods so avoid it for Phase 2 of the eating plan and only re-introduce it on an infrequent basis when you are feeling that your immune system is well enough to cope.

Q43) How can I stop Food Intolerance coming back?

A) The key causes of Food Intolerance are **repeated overexposure** to a particular food or food family. Hence, to stop this happening again, don't eat too much of one particular food or food family and don't eat it too often. Exactly the advice in Phase 3 – don't cheat too much and don't cheat too often. Try to have as much variety as possible in your food intake and eat different foods each day as much as you possibly can. If you get into the habit of having exactly the same breakfast, lunch or dinner every day, you are increasing the chances of developing a Food Intolerance.

Q44) Why do Food Intolerances vary from country to country?

A) The key cause of Food Intolerance is eating too much of any one substance too often. Hence the foods most often consumed in each country and in the largest quantities are the ones most likely to cause Food Intolerance. In Australia the foods eaten most of and most often are wheat and milk – the same as in the UK. In the US they are dairy foods, wheat, corn, eggs, soy, peanuts and sugar. In Taiwan they are rice and soya beans.

Hypoglycaemia – Chapter 11

Q45) What is Hypoglycaemia?

A) Hypoglycaemia is literally a Greek translation from "*hypo*" meaning 'under', "*glykis*" meaning 'sweet' and "*emia*" meaning 'in the blood together'. The three bits all put together mean low blood glucose.

Q46) What causes Hypoglycaemia?

A) The key cause of Hypoglycaemia is the consumption of refined carbohydrates. If you remember from Chapter 2, if you eat an apple your body normally releases the right amount of insulin to 'mop' up the glucose in your blood and to return your blood glucose level to normal. If you drink a carton of apple juice, your body thinks you have eaten, say, 20 apples and releases the amount of insulin needed to cope with lots of apples. Because you haven't eaten lots of apples there is an excess of insulin in your body and this will have the effect of lowering your blood glucose level below normal. You are now in a state of Hypoglycaemia, by definition, as your blood glucose level is low.

Q47) How do I know if I have Hypoglycaemia?

A) Hypoglycaemia can be diagnosed with a glucose tolerance test, which involves a series of blood tests being taken, after a glucose drink has been drunk, to measure the person's tolerance for sugar. This test is rarely performed at the suggestion of a doctor and it may be difficult to persuade your doctor to refer you for one.

One of the best tests, much more available than a glucose tolerance test, is to follow the Phase 1 eating plan in this book for five days. If you have stable energy levels, a clear head and your other symptoms of Hypoglycaemia have subsided then you can be sure that Hypoglycaemia was a problem for you.

The symptoms of Hypoglycaemia include the following:

Head – headaches; dizziness; blurred vision; feeling of 'sleepwalking'; feeling unreal; feeling 'spaced out'.

Women – PMT.

Blood Glucose – hungry between meals; irritable or moody before meals; shaky when hungry; faintness when food is not eaten; irregular pulse before and after eating; headaches late morning; waking in the early hours and not being able to get back to sleep; abnormal cravings for sweets or caffeine; eating sweets increases hunger; excessive appetite; instant sugar 'high' followed by fatigue; chilly feeling after eating.

Mental – anxiety; depression; irritability; lethargy; memory problems; loss of concentration; moodiness; nightmares; mental 'sluggishness'; *"get up and go"* has got up and gone.

Other – dramatic fluctuations in weight from one day to the next; exhaustion; feeling of being unable to cope; constant fatigue; excessive thirst; easy weight gain.

Q48) How does Hypoglycaemia cause food cravings?

A) This is a really simple one. As soon as your blood glucose level falls below normal, your body will cry out for food. It will crave any food but, most likely, sweet foods to get your blood glucose level back up again. When your hands are shaking, you feel a bit sweaty, a bit light headed or even faint in extreme cases, this is your body begging you to eat. You reach for a confectionery bar and immediately feel better, almost euphoric, as your blood glucose level shoots up. However, the confectionery bar is alien to your pancreas, so your body overproduces insulin, your blood glucose level falls below normal again and the cravings continue.

Q49) How can you treat Hypoglycaemia?

A) This is pretty simple too – stop eating refined carbohydrates. You should switch to a low carbohydrate diet for a few days to confirm the diagnosis (Phase 1) and to see just how well you can feel and then continue to eat only **un**refined (whole-meal) carbohydrates (Phase 2).

Q50) How can I stop Hypoglycaemia coming back?

A) Ideally keep the first rule of Phase 2 as a life-long way of eating – don't eat refined carbohydrates. You will still be able to eat rice, pasta, bread and all the things you may enjoy at the moment – but just have the brown, whole-meal version instead of the white refined version. Watch your consumption of all carbohydrates, even fruits, to see how much your body can tolerate without getting a blood glucose high and then low. You may find apples are fine, for example, but that tropical fruits are too sweet for you.

Q51) What if I have none of the conditions, or only one or two of them?

A) The fewer conditions you have the better for you. You may have read this book in time and caught things before they get too bad. You may have none of the conditions and are craving food just because you have been calorie counting and, therefore, need more petrol in your tank. If you only have Candida then you will need to avoid yeast, sugar and vinegar in Phase 2 but you may find you are able to tolerate wheat for example. If you only have a particular Food Intolerance, such as milk, then avoid that food in Phase 2. If you don't crave any particular foods (which would suggest Food Intolerance) and you don't think Candida is a problem for you but you are getting strong swings in your blood glucose level then it may be just Hypoglycaemia that you need to think about. The fewer conditions you have, the more options for food you have in Phase 2.

This Eating Plan

Q52) What should I eat?

A) In Phase 1 – for five days – you should eat meat, fish, eggs, tofu (if you are tolerant to soy products), quorn, Natural Live Yoghurt (NLY), any salad, any vegetables (except potatoes and mushrooms) and some brown rice (2oz dry weight for meat and/or fish eaters and up to 6oz for vegetarians – per day).

In Phase 2 – for as long as you need to reach your natural weight – the rules are 1) Don't eat refined carbohydrates, 2) Don't eat anything that will perpetuate any of the three conditions that you are suffering from and 3) Don't eat fat and carbohydrate at the same meal.

In Phase 3 – life-long – keep to the rules of Phase 2 for most of the time but you can then eat what you want **almost** when you want provided you 1) don't cheat too much, 2) don't cheat too often and 3) be alert and stay in control.

Q53) How much should I eat?

A) In Phase 1 – as much as you want. Don't count calories and don't go hungry.

In Phase 2 – as much as you want. Don't count calories and don't go hungry.

In Phase 3 – as much as you can get away with. Don't cheat too much or too often and look out for any return of the cravings. At the first sight of food addiction go back to Phase 2 or even Phase 1 for a short, sharp correction.

Overall – eat as much as you like so long as you don't count calories. In the first few days eat as much as you like and as much as you can to make sure you aren't hungry when the cravings are at their highest. You are better to eat massive vegetable dishes and as much fat/protein as you want during these first five days just to ensure that you don't give in to the cravings. You are likely to find that you actually don't fancy very much in the first few days as you will be eating foods that you have little interest in – i.e. the foods that you **don't** crave.

As the cravings subside in Phase 2 you should start listening to your body as it will tell you when it is hungry (before it was just telling you it wanted a food to which you were addicted). When your natural appetite emerges, eat as much as your body is telling you to. If you need several pieces of fruit upon wakening, a large bowl of porridge for breakfast, cheese for a mid morning snack, a large portion of protein and salad with oily dressing for lunch, an apple mid afternoon and a large portion of brown rice and vegetarian chilli for dinner with strawberries for pudding, then have this!

Q54) What should I have for breakfast?

A) In Phase 1 – eggs, bacon & eggs, Natural Live Yoghurt, omelette, steak, fish – whatever you fancy from the 'allowed' list.

In Phase 2 – a fat breakfast, or fruit when you wake up followed by a carbohydrate breakfast. Carbohydrate breakfasts can be whole-meal toast (sugar free) or any sugar free cereal – no fat. Fat breakfasts can be eggs, bacon & eggs etc. – no carbohydrate.

In Phase 3 – it is a really good idea to follow Phase 2 and get the day off to a good start – save the 'cheating' to later.

Q55) What should I have for main meals?

A) Phase 1 – meat, fish, tofu, quorn, eggs, Natural Live Yoghurt, brown rice, vegetables and salad – lots of options are offered in Chapter 13.

Phase 2 – either a carbohydrate meal or a fat meal – lots of options are offered in Chapter 14.

Phase 3 – the simplest 'rule' to drop in Phase 3 is not mixing fat and carbohydrate. This will allow you to have whole-meal sandwiches, baked potatoes & fillings, 'normal' restaurant meals etc. This, however, will need watching closely as your body will store fat if carbohydrates are available at the same time. If you find you are putting weight back on then go back to not mixing fat and carbohydrate – or mix them, but not too much and not too often. Remember Phase 3 is all about you being in control and getting the balance between eating what you want and being the weight you want.

Q56) Why do I have to stop eating the foods I most like?

A) Because these are the foods you most crave and you crave foods that are causing you problems – this is the real irony of Candida, Food Intolerance and Hypoglycaemia. The foods you don't crave are not causing you problems. This is why meat, fish, eggs, vegetables, brown rice and Natural Live Yoghurt are generally OK for anyone – they are hardly ever the subject of cravings.

Q57) What should I have for snacks?

A) Phase 1 – any protein snacks (hardboiled eggs, NLY, slices of meat etc).
    Phase 2 – protein snacks as above or fruit.
    Phase 3 – ideally protein snacks, 70+% cocoa chocolate, fruit and whole-meal cereal bars. However, you can eat anything that you want provided you follow the cheating guidelines!

Q58) What should I drink?

A) Ideally lots of water and herbal teas at every phase of the eating plan.
    Phase 1 – water, herbal teas, decaffeinated coffee (no milk).
    Phase 2 – water, herbal teas, decaffeinated coffee, milk (if you are tolerant to milk), an occasional glass of wine with the main meal (if you are tolerant to yeast and grapes and Candida is not a problem for you). (Also – remember the caffeine exception in Chapter 14 – if you must have a cup of coffee or tea to start the day then do. The key thing is to stick to the eating plan).
    Phase 3 – what you want but don't cheat too much, too often and be alert and stay in control.

Q59) How long should I leave between a fat meal and a carbohydrate meal?

A) The general guideline is three to four hours because this is how long it normally takes for food to be digested. You should achieve this naturally by having three meals a day. Take care if you are having snacks between meals as you could have a 'fat' snack mid morning and then a carbohydrate meal at lunchtime before the fat snack is out of the way. You will need to allow for snacks in these time guidelines, therefore, and not eat a carbohydrate meal within three to four hours of a fat snack, or vice versa.

Q60) How do I start this eating plan?

A) Start with Phase 1, for five days, as soon as you a) have read this book, b) know why you crave food, c) are prepared to stop counting calories and d) are prepared to start a journey that will change your life. Don't come up with excuses for not starting it. Every day that you delay, your cravings will get worse and the battle will be that much harder when you do start it.

Q61) When do I move on to different phases?

A) Move on to Phase 2 after five days unless you have a big problem with Candida and need to stay on Phase 1 longer. Phase 1 can be followed safely and healthily for some time but it is quite restrictive so the idea is to widen your food choices as soon as possible. You can dip back into Phase 1 and do another five day burst whenever you feel like it (as a detox or as an extra weight loss boost).

Q62) How long do I have to stay on the eating plan?

A) We advise five days for Phase 1 (you can do this for longer), as long as you like for Phase 2 (some people may choose this for life and others may like the thought of 'managed cheating' in Phase 3).

Q63) What do I do if I eat something that is not good for me?

A) Don't start a binge. Get back on track. Don't let one small slip ruin all the efforts you have made. To minimise the damage done, drink lots of water to enable your body to detox more easily. If the thing that you have eaten is something that will cause a sharp rise (and fall) in blood glucose level then watch out for the fall and don't let this lead to further cravings. Just as you feel your blood glucose high is wearing off, eat a piece of fruit or some whole-meal carbohydrates (e.g. a sugar free oat biscuit) to help your blood glucose level rise gently when it is about to crash down.

If what you have eaten triggers cravings, you may need to return to Phase 1 until the cravings subside again.

Finally, try to learn from what has happened. Why did you eat something that wasn't good for you? Have the cravings returned? If so, why? Is Candida still a problem for you? Are you in the first few days of Phase 1 and the cravings are unbearable? If so, re-read the motivational section and see how you can get through the five days next time. Unless you plan to exist, not live, you will have to tackle this some time so do it now. Are you in Phase 3 and have you been cheating too much and/or too often? If so return to Phase 2 until you feel in control again and cut back on your cheating next time. It really is trial and error until you know what **you** can get away with.

Q64) I want more rules – can I have a day to day eating plan?

A) I have tried to minimise the rules as so many diet books have too many rules to read, let alone follow. The idea of 1) Don't eat refined carbohydrates 2) Don't eat anything that will perpetuate any of the three conditions that you are suffering from and 3) Don't eat fat and carbohydrate at the same meal – is to give you really simple headlines that you can get ingrained into your way of thinking and follow any time, anywhere.

You can spend some time during Phase 1 coming up with an eating plan for yourself if you are one of those people who likes eating plans all spelled out day by day. If I devise one for you, you are bound to not like some of the foods on the list and then you will find excuses not to stick to it.

Pick the foods that you enjoy, that are within your budget, that you know you can get in the supermarket at this time of year and make a one week menu plan which you can then repeat week after week. Some people like this kind of routine – I'm not one of them. The Rotation Eating Plan in Chapter 17 is as close as we get to a prescribed eating plan in this book.

An example day's eating for Phase 2 could be as follows:
- First thing – fruit (a great cleanser first thing in the morning) – as much as you like.
- Breakfast – sugar free, natural porridge oats with skimmed or semi skimmed milk (or water if you are intolerant to milk) – as much as you like.
- Lunch – any meat, fish, tofu, quorn or eggs with any vegetables or salad; berries & Natural Live Yoghurt for afters.
- Dinner – brown rice with stir-fry vegetables or whole-wheat pasta and tomato sauce; an occasional glass of wine.
- Snacks – fruit or cheese if you must have something in between meals.

261

Q65) How healthy is this eating plan?

A) This eating plan essentially tells you not to eat refined carbohydrates. These are foods with a lot of the nutrients and goodness removed so we are actually much better off and much healthier for not eating these. This eating plan lets you eat all natural foods which are full of nutrients like fruit, vegetables, salad, meat, fish, dairy products, whole grains. It is very healthy indeed.

What will happen on this Eating Plan?

Q66) How will I feel?

A) In Phase 1 you could feel quite unwell – like having a mild flu. You may have headaches from food addiction withdrawal. You may feel lethargic and you may have little interest in the foods that are allowed, as what you really want are the others foods – the ones that you crave. You are likely to have unbelievable cravings but just take each day at a time, each hour at a time if necessary, and the cravings absolutely will subside. By the end of Phase 1 (for some people after just two to three days) you could start feeling fantastic – more mentally alert and clear headed than you have done for ages. You should notice your skin has a lovely natural colour, not the red, blotchy colour you get when you keep eating foods to which you are intolerant. Your eyes will sparkle and you will sleep better than you have done for ages (not a carbohydrate induced stupor from which you wake feeling sluggish).

In Phase 2 you should feel great. The cravings will be barely noticeable. You may still **want** your previous favourites but you won't have an overwhelming craving for them as you have had in the past. You really will be able to take them or leave them. Don't be fooled too early into thinking you can eat them again and not have the cravings return. You need to get to your natural weight, and realise how wonderful life is when you are slim and energetic and free from food addiction, before you can make an informed choice about whether or not to have the 'forbidden' foods again.

In Phase 3 you should feel free! The key thing about Phase 3 is that you have the freedom to eat what you want **almost** when you want and you will have the tools to stay in control. You will find that you get to the point where you are making sober and informed choices. When you are genuinely not craving refined carbohydrates you will find it easy to reject them in favour of foods that fill you up and make you feel good. For the first time in your life, you will control your eating, your eating won't control you.

Q67) How much effort will this be?

A) How does the well known saying go? – 'you don't get something for nothing'. If you really want to be slim, more than you want to eat, you now have the knowledge and tools to achieve this. You know you just have to stop the cravings and then your eating can be back in your control. Phase 1 will be an effort but it is just five days long. How long is that? Nothing in terms of the rest of your life. Put all your remaining willpower into those five days and your cravings will be manageable by the end of Phase 1.

Phase 2 should be not much effort at all. It will almost seem unfair that you are not hungry, that you are eating healthy foods, feeling full of life and energy and still losing weight.

Phase 3 is as much or as little effort as you make it. If you don't cheat too much or too often you will find your cravings easy to manage and you will love the freedom of being able to cheat and have others wonder how you stay so slim.

What you will find is that if you cheat too much, or too often, the cravings will return and then you will have to go back to where you are now to fight the food addiction and cravings that return. You will then need to return to Phase 1 or Phase 2 to get back in control.

Q68) What will be the benefits?

A) Almost too many to list:
- Feeling wonderful that you are nourishing and nurturing your body rather than stuffing and starving it,
- Feeling high energy and a real zest for life,
- Reaching and maintaining a healthy weight,
- Having sparkling eyes, clear skin, sleeping well and feeling good,
- Having a strengthened immune system enabling you to resist infections, colds and flu that others are susceptible to,
- Feeling you control food rather than that food controls you,
- No longer feeling afraid of food, no longer avoiding social events because you are concerned about food or your weight.

Q69) What if I don't do something?

A) Sadly food addiction is not a steady state that you can decide to tackle in weeks, months or years time. Every day that you continue to feed Candida, eat foods to which you are intolerant, or upset your blood glucose level, you are making your food addiction, cravings and health worse. The longer you leave it before tackling your food addiction the worse it will get. I cannot urge you strongly enough – **tackle it now** – before it gets any worse and, therefore, even harder to tackle. Remember the vicious and virtuous circles? The choice really is yours – do nothing and it will get worse and worse until you can barely get out of bed and you may loathe yourself and your size even more than you do now. Do something and the rest of your life starts now.

Eating Plans in general

Q70) What are the characteristics of a successful eating plan?

A) The five characteristics of a successful eating plan are:
1) It must work and not just in the short term. It must work in the long term, i.e. it must help you reach your natural weight and stay there.
2) It must be practical – a real eating plan for the real world. No working out grams of protein or counting calories or carbohydrates – some simple rules that you can follow at home, at work or at play as part of your busy lifestyle.
3) It must be a long term way of eating, something you can stick to and not something you go on and then go off leading to life-long weight fluctuations.
4) It must be healthy and deliver the nutrients you need for healthy living.
5) It must be enjoyable and not take away eating as a pleasure in life.

Q71) Why don't fad diets work?

A) They don't meet any of the characteristics of a successful diet. They work in the very short term and only then if you can stick to them.

Q72) Atkins works for me…

A) If Atkins works for you – great. (Why are you reading this book, by the way?) If you have found any diet that works for you then stick with it – you are in a real minority. If, however, Atkins works for you but you still have insatiable cravings that you are constantly fighting, or you would give anything just to have an apple or a banana, then try going onto Phase 2. You don't have to give up fruits and whole grains. Nutty brown rice with char-grilled or stir-fried vegetables is a joy to eat and it is good for you. Whole-wheat pasta with an Italian tomato sauce is delicious. Fruit is one of the best natural things on the planet. There is no reason to avoid all carbohydrates – just refined carbohydrates.

Q73) What about the cabbage soup diet? Liquid diets? Etc

A) What about them? They are all fad diets, they don't work in the long term, they are not healthy, they are not enjoyable, they are nearly impossible to stick to, they do not re-educate you or change your eating habits. They have not worked for you in the past and they will not work for you in the future. If you really want to drop a clothes size in five days, do Phase 1.

Other Questions – General

Q74) What about alcohol?

A) You can't drink alcohol in Phase 1. If the thought of giving up alcohol for five days fills you with horror, you have a drink problem! It may well be that this is one of the products you crave and, as alcohol is made up of sugar, yeast, wheat, hops and many other substances that are commonly not tolerated, you may be craving alcohol for good reason. You may find that your craving for alcohol is also driving your cravings for sweets, bread, pasta, pizza and so on.

In Phase 2 you can drink an **occasional** glass of (ideally red) wine with your main meal but beer and spirits must still be avoided. Don't have wine every day and avoid it more often than not in Phase 2 – save your cheating for Phase 3.

In Phase 3 you may decide to use your cheating entirely for alcohol but watch carefully for any sign that you are craving alcohol. Test yourself against the four characteristics of food addiction – if you find that you are having the substance every day, need more of it to have the same effect, feel good when you have it and bad when you don't – you are hooked again.

Q75) What about vegetarianism?

A) There is a whole chapter on vegetarianism. The bottom line is that you can follow this eating plan as a vegetarian. Phase 1 is quite limited, but Phase 2 and 3 are fine for vegetarians – I have been one for several years. The real problem would be for vegans as this eating plan would be very restrictive for vegans. If you are an overweight vegan with food addiction you may seriously need to think about whether or not your health is suffering with your commendable principles. Is there any way you can compromise a bit? Free range eggs, for example, or organic milk?

Q76) What about exercise?

A) Exercise is good for you full stop. Think of it as part of your overall plan to be healthy and fit and to lead an active and energetic life. The only bad reason for exercising is to increase your need for calories! Exercise can actually lower your blood glucose level so watch out for hunger pangs after working out and have a piece of fruit and lots of water close by to stop cravings for other things.

Q77) Why are more women than men obese?

A) Remember cravings lead to overeating and overeating leads to overweight. Women are more likely than men to do the one thing that alone will make them crave food and that is calorie counting. Women are also more likely than men to have the three conditions that also cause food cravings. They are more likely than men to have Candida, as the woman's body is a more natural breeding group for the parasite and because women tend to eat low fat, high carbohydrate foods. Women are more likely to have Food Intolerance because, by counting calories, they restrict their intake of food and tend to stick to the same low calorie, low fat foods every day. Women are more likely than men to suffer Hypoglycaemia, again because they count calories and eat more carbohydrate whereas men tend to eat more fat and protein.

Q78) Why are more Americans than French overweight?

A) The French eat fat and shun sugar. They eat hardly any cakes, biscuits and refined carbohydrates but they do eat lots of meat, fish, fat, butter, cheese and cream and so on. The Americans shun fat and eat lots of sugar and refined carbohydrates as a result. The average American counts calories. The average French person eats real food as a part of real meals three times a day. The best proof that this eating plan works is to look at the French nation vs. America. The French eat fat and are thin. The Americans eat 'thin' (low fat) and are fat! Slim Americans, like movie stars and pop stars, either starve themselves on a regular basis to stay slim or they follow a low carbohydrate diet.

Q79) What is a natural weight?

A) A natural weight is the weight your body will reach at the end of Phase 2 i.e. when you are eating natural, healthy, **un**refined foods in the quantities that you need to avoid feeling hungry. It will be the weight that you find you can stay at easily in Phase 3 provided that you don't cheat too much or too often. You will only tend to dip below your natural weight if you are ill and genuinely lose your appetite. You will go above it if you cheat too much, too often. If you are 5ft, 4" and you want to be 100lb this is not a healthy goal and this will not be your natural weight. You may, however, find that 115-120lb is a natural weight range for you and you will be a slim, 'small clothes size', person at this weight. Don't be unrealistic with your goal weight, therefore, and don't think too much about your weight as you embark on this programme. The key goal is to stop cravings and doing this will stop the overeating and your weight will then tend towards its natural level quickly and easily.

Q80) So what happens now?

A) Read Part 9 for that final inspirational boost and then go for it!

PART 9

POSITIVE THINKING

MOTIVATIONAL THOUGHTS
TO CHANGE YOUR EATING FOR EVER

PART 9

POSITIVE THINKING

You now know that you overeat when all you want is to be slim because you have addict-like food cravings. You have these cravings because of one thing that you are doing, calorie counting, and because of one, or all, of three conditions that you may have – Candida, Food Intolerance and Hypoglycaemia. All of these are closely linked together and they are also linked to and caused by stress, modern medication and modern processed food.

Calorie counting directly causes cravings as your body will tell you to give it the energy (calories) that it needs. Candida drives you to crave sugary, yeasty and vinegary foods. Food Intolerance drives you to crave any food to which you are intolerant – this can literally be any food or drink from eggs to alcohol. Hypoglycaemia drives you to crave refined carbohydrates as your blood glucose level lurches from high to low on an hourly basis.

The key to overcoming overeating is to overcome cravings. You have failed so many times before because of these cravings. Stop counting calories; follow the strategies in this book to overcome Candida, Food Intolerance and Hypoglycaemia and you can free yourself from food cravings. When you are free from food cravings you will have a choice as to what you want to eat and when you want to eat it. Right now you do not have that choice – you are not greedy or weak willed. You are a food addict and you need to go 'cold turkey' on some foods just like a drug addict needs to go 'cold turkey' on their addictive substance.

You will succeed this time because you now have the power of knowledge. You know why you have failed before – because of the cravings. You know what you have been craving and why. You know that the cravings have come from calorie counting, Candida, Food Intolerance and Hypoglycaemia. You know that you have to eliminate the offending foods from your diet and watch the cravings disappear in literally days. You also know not to starve yourself, or to let yourself go hungry, as this is the surest way to slip up in the future.

This is the good news. The bad news is that there are now no excuses. You know why you overeat. You know how to stop it. You know that the only person who can control your eating is you. If you really do want to be slim for life then put all the willpower you undoubtedly do have into fighting food cravings. It won't be easy but nothing worth having ever is. Furthermore, I can promise you two things:

1) It will be worth it. Your health is the most important thing that you have in life – without it you have nothing. You must nurture, nourish and treat your body well rather than starve and stuff it and make yourself ill.

2) It will be easier than you think. You cannot imagine life without certain foods right now because you are addicted to them. In as few as five days, however, you could dramatically reduce that addiction. Every day that you nourish your body and avoid the foods that are harming it is another day nearer the healthy, slim you.

I know how it feels to be where you are now and I know how it feels to be where I am now. I would love every unhappy, overweight, food addict to be happy, slim and healthy and to be able to get on with something infinitely more important than food – life!

I wish you the very best in your journey and I will leave you with some thoughts that I sincerely hope will inspire you along the way:

Q1) WHO is going to change your life?
A) You are. It's up to you.

Q2) WHEN are you going to change your life?
A) Now! Unless you plan to be overweight for your entire life you've got to start sometime, so do it now. Every day that you continue to feed your food addiction it gets worse. The longer you leave this the harder it gets, so do it now.

Q3) HOW will you change your life?
A) By stopping food cravings because it is cravings that make you overeat when all you want is to be slim.

Q4) WHY are you going to change your life?
A) Because you only have one life. You don't intend to waste another day overweight and addicted to food.

PART 10

RECIPES

QUICK & EASY MENUS FOR ALL PHASES OF THE EATING PLAN

PART 10

Recipes

My husband is the cook in our household so many thanks to him for this section of the book. You will notice that our recipes are quick, simple and they all use natural ingredients. All but one recipe is sugar free (the indulgent chocolate mousse is the one exception which is for Phase 3 only). Most of them are also wheat free (any pasta dish can be made with rice pasta). We work in both metric and imperial measurements (we're from the measurement changeover age group) so we have put a conversion table in below to help you. We have also included an oven temperature conversion table to help you with your own kitchen stove.

If these recipes leave you wanting more, we highly recommend two books called "*Cooking without*" and "*Cooking Without for Vegetarians*" by Barbara Cousins, which are quite excellent for people suffering from Candida, Food Intolerance and Hypoglycaemia.

Weight/Measurement Conversions
Metric to Imperial:

1 litre	=	1.75 pints
1 kg	=	2.2lb
100g	=	3.5oz

Imperial to Metric:

1 pint/16fl oz	=	568ml (sometimes known as 2 cups)
1oz	=	28.4g
1lb	=	454g

Oven Temperature Conversions

FAHRENHEIT	CENTIGRADE	GAS MARK	DESCRIPTION
225 – 275 f	110 – 135 c	0 – 1	Very Cool
300 – 325 f	150 – 165 c	2 – 3	Cool
350 – 375 f	175 – 190 c	4 – 5	Moderate
400 – 425 f	200 – 220 c	6 – 7	Hot
450 – 475 f	230 – 245 c	8 – 9	Very Hot

Here are the recipes that were promised in Part 4 of this book:

Breakfasts

FAT OPTIONS	CARBOHYDRATE OPTIONS
- Full English breakfast (C, H, P1) - Scrambled eggs * (C, H, P1,V) - Omelettes * (C, H, P1,V)	- Fruit platters (C, H, V)
* Made without milk so that they can be suitable for Phase 1 and for people with Food Intolerance.	No more than 1-2 portions of fruit per day if you have Candida and/or Hypoglycaemia.

Full English Breakfast
This low/zero carbohydrate meal ensures that barely any insulin is produced so, if insulin isn't there, then the fat can't be stored.
Choose from:
- Grilled or fried bacon (avoid smoked bacon to keep Candida at bay). Bacon can be fried in butter or olive oil.
- Eggs as you like them (provided of course that you are tolerant to eggs) – scrambled, fried (in butter), poached etc.
- Steak or any other pure meat if you fancy it.
- A few mushrooms and tomatoes fried in butter (no mushrooms if Candida is a problem for you and only a couple of tomatoes as they are carbohydrates).

Avoid:
- Sausages as they are almost always packed with other ingredients.
- All carbohydrates other than tomatoes or mushrooms.
- All sauces e.g. tomato sauce, ketchup, brown sauce etc. – as these are all laden with sugar and often other refined carbohydrates too.

Scrambled Eggs (No Milk)
- Crack 2 eggs per person into a mixing bowl and beat with a fork, or an electric whisk, until fluffy.
- Melt a knob of butter in a frying pan and add the whisked eggs.
- Continually stir the eggs in the pan (with a wooden spoon) until they become the consistency that you like (experiment with different cooking times depending on whether you like them soft and runny or firmer). The longer you cook them the firmer they will get.

Omelettes (No Milk)
- Crack 2 or 3 eggs per person into a mixing bowl and beat with a fork, or an electric whisk, until fluffy.
- Add about ½ teaspoon of mixed herbs and some freshly ground black pepper.
- Melt a knob of butter in a frying pan and add the whisked eggs.
- Cook slowly until the mixture becomes firm. (You can tilt the pan to move the mixture around to make sure it covers the pan but don't stir it or you will end up with scrambled eggs).

This can be served with a mixed salad for a main meal.

For a flavoured Omelette, add some of your favourite ingredients to the whisked eggs before pouring them into the frying pan. The classic options are ham, cheese and mushrooms.

Fruit Platters

Ideally get an oversized plate/platter (a normal plate will be fine if you don't have a giant one).

Buy a good selection of ripe, fresh, fruit in season and get chopping. Leave any edible skins on and chop all the fruit so that you just have to dive in with fingers and enjoy. This is a really satisfying meal and seems a lot more filling than when you just eat pieces of fruit on their own. You can add a couple of spoonfuls of low fat cottage cheese or low fat Natural Live Yoghurt in the middle of the platter for a filling dip.

Tropical Fruit Platter:

Pineapple, mango, melon, paw paw, papaya, banana, sharon fruit, star fruit, kiwi fruit and grapes – whatever you can find in the grocery store.

Berry Fruit Platter:

Strawberries, raspberries, blueberries and blackberries – again whatever you can find.

Stone Fruit Platter:

Nectarines, peaches, plums and apricots.

Citrus Fruit Platter:

Orange segments, grapefruit segments, kumquats, satsumas and clementines.

Staple Fruit Platter:

Available all year round – sliced apples, sliced pears, grapes and bananas.

FAT OPTIONS	CARBOHYDRATE OPTIONS
No recipes in this section	- Char-grilled vegetables with balsamic or olive oil dressing (C, H, P1, V) - A selection of soups (C, H, P1,V)

Char-grilled Vegetables

- Brush a baking tray with olive oil.
- Place a selection of sliced or diced vegetables (aubergine/eggplant, courgette/zucchini, onions, mushrooms, peppers and carrots work well) on the baking tray and brush the vegetables with olive oil.
- Roast them in a medium oven until the vegetables are blackened and soft to a fork touch (approximately 30 minutes).
- Flavour with balsamic vinegar (not in Phase 1, or if you have Candida) or extra olive oil if desired.
- Add a few pine nuts and/or a small grating of Parmesan cheese for extra taste.
  Vegetable kebabs can be done with the same vegetables on a skewer on a BBQ or roasted in the oven.

Vegetable Soup (Serves 6)

This is a real winter warming soup and it feels hearty and filling.
  You will need:

- 1 large onion finely chopped,
- 1 clove garlic finely chopped,
- 1kg (2.2lb) of root vegetables (carrots, parsnips, swede, potatoes, and turnips) chopped into 1 inch cubes,
- Olive oil for cooking (approximately 2 tablespoons),
- 1.5 pints of vegetable stock (home-made or from a sugar free stock cube).

What you do with all this:

- Heat the olive oil in a large pan.
- Fry the onion and garlic lightly until the onion becomes transparent.
- Add all the vegetables and give them a good stir.
- Add the vegetable stock and bring everything to the boil.
- Reduce the heat and simmer lightly for about 30 minutes or until the vegetables are cooked.
- Turn off the heat and allow to cool for 5 minutes before serving.
- Leave chunky, or use a hand held blender to blend the mixture until smooth.

Carrot & Coriander Soup (Serves 6)

This exotic sounding soup is simple and quick to make and is absolutely delicious. It can be served as a meal on its own or as a starter at a dinner party. This does have a small amount of fat (cream & butter) but that's OK with coloured vegetables on occasions.

You will need:
- 1 large onion finely chopped,
- 1 garlic clove crushed,
- A knob of butter,
- 1lb of carrots, ¾ thinly sliced and ¼ grated,
- 1.75 pints (1 litre) vegetable stock,
- A handful of freshly chopped coriander,
- 150ml (approximately a quarter of a pint) of single cream,

What you do with all this:
- Melt the butter in a large pan.
- Fry the onion and garlic lightly until the onion becomes transparent.
- Add the chopped carrots and give the mix a good stir.
- Add the vegetable stock and bring to the boil.
- Reduce the heat and simmer lightly for about 30 minutes or until the carrots are cooked.
- Turn off the heat and allow the mixture to cool for 10 minutes.
- Use a hand held blender to blend the mixture until smooth.
- Stir in the grated carrots and coriander and then the cream.
- Serve with a sprinkle of chopped coriander.
  This soup can be cooked in advance and re-heated as required.

Roasted Tomato Soup (Serves 6)

It takes a bit of time to pre grill the tomatoes in this recipe but it really is worth it. The taste of the roasted vegetables makes the whole soup really special.

You will need:
- 3lb of medium tomatoes (yes 3lb),
- 3 cloves garlic, crushed,
- 2 large onions, sliced,
- 1 medium fennel, sliced,
- 2 sticks celery, chopped,
- Olive oil for cooking,

What you do with all this:
- Cut the tomatoes in half and put them on baking trays lightly covered in olive oil.
- Place them under a very hot grill for 10 minutes. (You may need to do them in batches if you don't have lots of baking trays and a large grill).
- Transfer them all to a large saucepan once they have been grilled.
- Put the olive oil into a large frying pan and lightly fry the onions, garlic, fennel and celery until the onions begin to soften.
- Then, transfer all the fried ingredients onto a baking dish and place them at the top of a medium oven, gas mark 4-5 for 30 minutes.
- Pour all the fried & oven baked vegetables onto the grilled tomatoes in the saucepan and mix well.
- Use a hand held blender to blend the mixture until smooth.
- Warm everything in the saucepan (not quite to boiling point) and serve immediately.

Gazpacho Soup (Serves 6)

This is the easiest recipe for this classic summer soup that you'll ever find.

You will need:
- 1 large cucumber, peeled and chopped,
- 1 large onion, peeled and chopped,
- 1 red pepper & 1 green pepper, de-seeded and chopped,
- 1 litre (1.75 pints) of tomato juice, chilled,
- Juice of 1 lemon,
- A tablespoon of sunflower oil,

What you do with all this:
- In batches, put handfuls of the ingredients in a blender (liquidiser) and blend until smooth.
- In the final batch, add the lemon juice and sunflower oil.
- Chill for two hours before serving.

Main Meals – Main Courses

FAT OPTIONS	CARBOHYDRATE OPTIONS
- Salade niçoise (C, H, P1)	- Stir-fry vegetables (C, H, P1, V)
- Salmon niçoise (C, H, P1)	- 5 minute tomato sauce (C, H, V)
- Cheese sauce for Cheesy leeks or cauliflower cheese (C, H, V)	- Vegetarian chilli and brown rice (C, H, V)
- Aubergine/eggplant bake (C, H, V)	- Whole-wheat cous-cous and char-grilled vegetables (C, H, V)
- Aubergine/eggplant boats (C, H, V)	- Whole-wheat cous-cous and chick peas in coriander sauce (C, H, V)
- Roast leg of lamb with rosemary & vegetables (C, H, P1)	- Butternut squash curry & brown rice (C, H, P1, V)
- Roast chicken with garlic or lemon (C, H, P1)	- Lentil moussaka (C, H, V)
- Four cheese salad (C, H, V)	- Roasted vegetables with pine nuts & Parmesan cheese (C, H, V)
	- Stuffed tomatoes (C, H, P1, V)
	- Stuffed peppers (C, H, P1, V)

Main Meals – Main Courses – Fat Options :

Salade Niçoise/Salmon Niçoise (Serves 1)
You will need:
- ½ iceberg lettuce,
- 6 cherry tomatoes,
- 2 inches of cucumber,
- 1 cup green beans,
- 1 egg,
- Char-grilled tuna steak or tinned tuna,
- French salad dressing,
- Salt & Pepper to taste,

What you do with all this:
- Chop the green beans into lengths of around an inch long. Cook them in boiling water until they are as soft or as crunchy as you like them.
- Hard boil an egg (you can do this in the same pan as the green beans).
- Chop the lettuce up quite finely and cover the plate with it.
- Slice the cherry tomatoes in two and place them around the edge of the plate.
- Dice the cucumber and sprinkle this over the lettuce, add the cooked green beans when they have cooled.

- Quarter the hard boiled egg and arrange it nicely around the plate.
- Add French dressing to taste (see the extras recipe section).
- Place the char-grilled tuna steak (cook raw tuna on the BBQ or on a skillet or just place it under a normal grill) or the tinned tuna in the middle of the plate.

TIP 1 – Salmon niçoise is becoming popular as an alternative to tuna. Just use a salmon steak or tinned salmon instead of tuna.

Cheese Sauce (Serves 2)
This sauce can be used to make either cauliflower cheese or cheesy leeks or any other cheese and vegetable dish. The recipe below uses cauliflower but pour the sauce over any vegetable you fancy.
You will need:
- 1 small cauliflower, quartered, or 4 small leeks,
- ½ pint milk,
- 1 egg, whisked,
- 3oz grated Cheddar cheese,

What you do with all this:
- Part cook the vegetables by lightly boiling or steaming them. Then place them in an oven-proof dish.
- In a saucepan, bring the milk to the boil then turn off the heat. Allow the milk to cool for 2 minutes then mix in the whisked egg.
- Add the grated cheese and stir continuously until the cheese has melted and you have a thick sauce.
- Pour over the cauliflower (or leeks), sprinkle with a little grated cheese and place in the oven, gas mark 4 for 20-30 minutes. Serve hot.

Aubergine/Eggplant Bake (Serves 4)

Aubergine/eggplant is a coloured vegetable so it does have a higher carbohydrate content than green vegetables. However, this still counts as a fat meal as the 1 aubergine/eggplant is a small part of the overall recipe.

- 1 aubergine/eggplant,
- 2 courgettes/zucchini,
- 1 red onion,
- 1 clove garlic finely chopped,
- 1 red pepper,
- 250g mozzarella,
- 100g Emmental (or other hard cheese like Edam or Cheddar),
- 2 tablespoons tomato puree (dissolved in 1 pint, 568ml, of vegetable stock),
- Pine nut kernels,
- Olive oil for cooking,

What you do with all this:
- Place 1 layer of vegetables in a baking dish (approximately 20 x 30 cm): first the red onion sliced into rings; then the courgettes/zucchini cut into 0.5cm thick slices and then the aubergine/eggplant cut into 0.5cm thick slices.
- Sprinkle the garlic on before adding further layers, in the above order, until all the vegetables are in the dish.
- Pour the tomato puree and vegetable stock over the vegetables and sprinkle a handful of pine nut kernels over everything.
- Cover the top layer of vegetables with a drizzle of olive oil.
- Slice the Mozzarella on top of the vegetables.
- Cut the red pepper into strips and lay it on top of the mozzarella.
- Grate the Emmental on top of everything.
- Bake in the oven on gas mark 4 for approximately an hour or until the cheese topping is crisp and brown.

Aubergine/Eggplant Boats (Serves 2 – 1 boat each)
You will need:
- 1 large aubergine/eggplant,
- 1 large onion (finely chopped),
- 1 clove garlic (crushed),
- 4 button mushrooms (finely chopped),
- 2 medium tomatoes (finely chopped),
- Salt & Pepper to taste,
- 100g Emmental (or other hard cheese like Edam or Cheddar),
- Olive oil for cooking,

What you do with all this:
- Cut the aubergine/eggplant in two lengthways. Scoop out the flesh of the aubergine/eggplant to leave two 'boats' made from the outside.
- Chop the aubergine/eggplant flesh finely and chop the other vegetables – onion, garlic, mushrooms and tomatoes.
- Heat a wok up with some olive oil in it until the olive oil is sizzling.
- Stir-fry the onions and garlic for a couple of minutes alone before adding the mushrooms, aubergine/eggplant and tomatoes. Add a little seasoning (salt & pepper) whilst cooking. Stir-fry all until they start to turn brown.
- Pour the stir-fried vegetables into the eggplant boats.
- Grate the Emmental on top.
- Bake in the oven on gas mark 4 for approximately an hour or until the cheese topping is crisp and brown.

Roast Leg of Lamb with Rosemary & Vegetables (Serves 4)
Place the leg of lamb in a large roasting dish and sprinkle with rosemary (fresh if possible). Add a handful of garlic cloves (unpeeled) and pop the lot in a hot oven (gas 5/6) and roast until cooked to your liking. As a guide, allow 30 minutes to start with and then add 15 minutes for each kg for a medium roast or 25-30 minutes/kg for a well done roast. Serve with a selection of freshly cooked vegetables or stir-fry. The garlic cooked this way becomes sweet and can be eaten with the meat.

Roast Chicken with Garlic or Lemon (Serves 4)

The simple roast chicken can be vastly improved by stuffing it with cloves of peeled garlic or fresh lemons. Allow 6-8 cloves of garlic or 1 whole lemon, cut in quarters, for a medium sized chicken.

Cook on gas mark 4 for 60-90 minutes. Cook 'up-side-down' for the first 30 minutes for the juices to penetrate the breast meat and then turn over. Serve with a selection of vegetables in the winter or a mixed salad in the summer.

4 Cheese Salad (Serves 1)

We eat salads almost every day, even in the winter, as the goodness found in a large plate of raw vegetables is hard to beat. In the winter combine them with a warm soup and you will find this compensates for the chill of the salad.

You will need:

- ¼ iceberg lettuce,
- 6 cherry tomatoes,
- 2 inches of cucumber,
- ¼ red pepper,
- 1 stick celery,
- Sprinkling of pine nuts (if you like),
- Olive oil or balsamic or our French salad dressing,
- Various cheese options (Blue Cheese, Cheddar, Cottage Cheese, Edam, Emmental, Feta, Parmesan),
- Salt & Pepper to taste,

What you do with all this:

- Chop the lettuce up quite finely and cover the plate with it.
- Slice the cherry tomatoes in two and place them around the edge of the plate.
- Dice the cucumber, celery and pepper and sprinkle this over the lettuce (sprinkle a few pine nuts on too if you like these).
- Add your chosen dressing over the salad base.
- Place 100g, or so, of cottage cheese in the middle of the plate.
- Add cubes of cheese (approx 1cm cube) to taste around the outside. Feta with balsamic and cottage cheese goes really well together, so do Cheddar, Emmental, Parmesan and cottage cheese.

Main Meals – Main Courses – Carbohydrate Options

Stir-fry Vegetables (Serves 2)

Stir-frying vegetables seals in their flavour and goodness and is a delicious meal in itself or can be served as an accompaniment to other dishes. The amount of vegetables can be varied to suit but, as a guide, allow approximately 200g of uncooked vegetables per person if serving as a main course. Don't worry if a dish looks too much, the vegetables will reduce dramatically in volume as you cook them.

You will need:

- A selection of chopped vegetables. Choose from cabbage (white, red and green), carrots, onions, peppers, chillies (add sparingly to taste), beans, baby sweet corn and anything else that you like,
- Sesame seed oil (or other flavoured oil),

What you do with all this:

- In a large wok, add a tablespoon of sesame seed oil and add all the chopped vegetables.
- Fry quickly on a high heat, stirring regularly, for about 5-8 minutes. When the vegetables start to soften, add ½ cupful of water, continuing to stir the vegetables. Add freshly ground black pepper to taste and a dash of Tabasco if you like a bite to your dishes.

For a variation on the above recipe, experiment with different oils (olive oil, groundnut oil) or add a handful of nuts with the water.

Serve with brown rice, quinoa or tofu.

5 Minute Home-made Tomato Sauce (Serves 2)

This is such a fantastic versatile sauce. It goes with pasta, spaghetti, quorn, vegetables and tofu or just about anything else you can think of. You will need:

- 1 large onion,
- 1 clove garlic,
- A 400g tin chopped tomatoes (check only tomatoes and citric acid are in the ingredients),
- 2 teaspoons of basil (ideally fresh),
- Salt & Pepper,
- Olive oil for cooking,

What you do with all this:
- Chop the garlic and onions finely.
- Heat a wok up until the olive oil is sizzling.
- Stir-fry the onion and garlic until slightly brown and then add the chopped tomatoes.
- Add the basil, salt & pepper and leave the sauce to simmer until some pasta is cooked (10-15 minutes).

TIP 1 this freezes well so make a big batch and put it into small tubs in the freezer to have quick pasta whenever you like.

TIP 2 if wheat is a problem for you, you can get rice pasta and corn pasta from health food shops, which looks and tastes just like wheat but without the side effects.

TIP 3 to make this a hot and spicy pasta sauce just buy some spicy olive oil and use this for cooking instead.

Vegetarian Chilli with Brown Rice (Serves 6)

This is a really filling dish and great for re-heating for quick meals.

You will need:

- 3lb of mixed vegetables cut into 1 inch cubes. Use carrots, courgette/zucchini, cauliflower, broccoli, and leeks – anything you like,
- 2 large onions, finely chopped,
- 1 clove garlic, crushed,
- 1 red pepper, deseeded and chopped into 1 inch squares,
- A 330ml tin of unsweetened kidney beans, drained,
- A 330ml tin chopped tomatoes,
- 2 medium chillies, deseeded and sliced,
- Chilli powder to taste (somewhere between 2 and 4 teaspoons),
- Olive oil for cooking,

What you do with all this:

- In a large saucepan or wok, heat the oil and lightly fry the onions for 10 minutes until transparent.
- Add the pepper and garlic and fry for a further 3-4 minutes.
- Then add all the mixed vegetables, including the drained kidney beans, tinned tomatoes and chillies and give it all a good stir.
- Stir in the chilli powder and then put the lid on the pan. Bring to the boil then reduce to simmering point and cook for 20-30 minutes or until the vegetables are cooked to your liking.
- Serve with brown rice.

Whole-wheat Cous-Cous & Chick Peas in Coriander Sauce (Serves 4)

(You can use the char-grilled vegetables recipe from the starters section and the cous-cous instructions below to make cous-cous with char-grilled vegetables).

You will need:

- 350g cous-cous,
- 1 pint (568 ml) vegetable stock,
- 1 tin (400g) chopped tomatoes,
- 1 tin (400g) chick peas, drained,
- Some finely chopped ginger,
- A handful of fresh coriander (or 2 tablespoons of dried),
- 1 large onion, finely chopped,
- 1 clove garlic, crushed,
- Olive oil for cooking,

What you do with all this:

- In a large saucepan, heat the oil and add the onion and garlic and lightly fry for about 10 minutes until the onion is transparent.
- Add the tin of tomatoes and chick peas and stir well.
- Add the ginger and coriander, put on the lid and simmer for 20-30 minutes.
- Meanwhile, put the cous-cous in a bowl and pour the vegetable stock over it. Cover with cling film and leave to stand for about 20-30 minutes.
- To serve, put a couple of spoons of cous-cous on a plate then spoon on the sauce. Garnish with some freshly chopped coriander.

Butternut Squash Curry (Serves 6)

This is a fantastic curry recipe to tempt even the most ardent carnivores away from meat. Butternut squash is like the meat of the vegetable kingdom.

You will need:
- 1kg (2lb) of mixed vegetables (like those in the vegetarian chilli) chopped into 1" squares,
- 1 large butternut squash, peeled, deseeded and cut into 1 inch squares,
- 3 large onions,
- 4 cloves garlic,
- 2 x 400ml tins of chopped tomatoes,
- 1 pint vegetable stock,
- 100g (3.5oz) block of creamed coconut,
- 2 teaspoons each of turmeric, cumin, paprika, coriander, chilli powder, curry powder (medium or hot depending on your preference),
- Olive oil for cooking,

What you do with all this:
- Heat the olive oil in a large saucepan and then lightly fry the onions and garlic for 15-20 minutes until transparent (do not brown).
- Transfer this mixture to a side dish then heat some more olive oil in the same pan and put in all the spices and lightly fry for 2-3 minutes.
- Put the onion mix back in the pan with the spices and mix thoroughly.
- Add the tinned tomatoes and vegetable stock and bring to the boil. Simmer for 5 minutes then remove from the heat and allow the mixture to cool slightly before blending it into a smooth mixture.
- Return the mixture to the heat and stir in the coconut block until it is completely dissolved.
- You now have a delicious curry sauce to which you can add all the vegetables. Put the lid on the saucepan and simmer gently until the vegetables are cooked to your liking (about 30 minutes).

Lentil Moussaka (Serves 6)

This dish is well worth the effort. It is tasty and impressive enough to serve at a dinner party and it is great to cook at the weekend and to take into work for lunches during the week (either cold or re-heated in a microwave). It can be served with roasted vegetables in the winter or with a Greek salad in the summer. This does have some fat in the topping but it is small relative to the rest of the ingredients so this is still a carbohydrate meal.

You will need:
- 2 large onions, finely chopped,
- 2 cloves of garlic, crushed,
- 1 red pepper, de-seeded and chopped into ½ inch pieces,
- 2 large aubergines/eggplants, diced into 1 inch cubes,
- 2 large (400g) tins of chopped tomatoes,
- 3 tablespoons of tomato puree,
- 4oz (113g) lentils (half green & half red),
- 1 pint vegetable stock,
- Olive oil for cooking,

For the topping:
- ½ pint low fat milk,
- A knob of butter,
- 1 egg,
- A small tub (250ml) of low fat ricotta cheese,
- Some grated Parmesan or Parmaggio cheese,

What you do with all this:
- Put some olive oil in a large frying pan or wok and lightly fry the onions for 10 minutes until they are transparent.
- Add the chopped pepper and fry for a further 5 minutes.
- Then add the crushed garlic and fry for a further 2-3 minutes.
- Transfer the mixture to a plate just to leave to one side for now.
- Add some more olive oil to the same frying pan or wok and fry the aubergines/eggplants until brown all over.
- Add back the fried onion, pepper and garlic and then add the tin of tomatoes, stock, tomato puree and lentils and give the mixture a good stir.
- Bring the whole mixture to boiling point and then reduce the heat to simmer for 10 minutes.
- Transfer the mixture to a large oven-proof dish; add the topping (see below) and then sprinkle with grated Parmesan cheese.

- Pop in a preheated oven (gas mark 5) for 45 minutes when the topping and Parmesan will be a nice brown. Allow to cool for 10 minutes before serving.

For the topping:
- Bring the milk and butter to the boil in a saucepan and then allow them to cool for 5 minutes.
- Add a whisked egg.
- Whisk the whole mixture and then whisk in the ricotta cheese. Add some freshly ground black pepper to taste.

Roasted vegetables with pine nuts & Parmesan (Serves 4)
This is a really simple and colourful dish which is especially nice in the winter when many different vegetables are readily available. There are a few nuts and a tiny bit of cheese in this carbohydrate recipe but not enough to make any real difference to your weight loss and they really add to the flavour.
You will need:
- 2lb of mixed vegetables cut into 2" cubes. Use Butternut squash, aubergine/eggplant and courgette/zucchini etc,
- 2 large onions, quartered,
- 1 clove garlic, crushed,
- 1 red pepper, deseeded and chopped into 1" squares,
- Olive oil for cooking,
- Grated Parmesan cheese,
- A sprinkling of pine nuts,
- Balsamic vinegar,

What you do with all this:
- In a large frying pan, heat the oil and lightly fry the onions and garlic for 2 minutes, then add all the other vegetables and stir-fry for a further 2 minutes.
- Put the mixture in a large oven-proof dish and roast in a hot oven, gas mark 6, for 30 minutes, stirring half way through.
- To serve, place a small amount of mixed green lettuce in an open, pasta type bowl and spoon on the roasted vegetables. Sprinkle with the grated Parmesan cheese and pine nuts and place under a very hot grill for 2 minutes just to melt the cheese. Dribble a small amount of balsamic vinegar around the edge of the bowl and serve immediately.

Stuffed Peppers/Tomatoes (Serves 4)

This can be done with either peppers or large tomatoes. The recipe below uses peppers as an example.

You will need:
- 4 peppers (red or green), deseeded, keeping the tops intact,
- 1 medium onion, finely chopped,
- 1 clove garlic, crushed,
- 4 medium sized mushrooms, finely chopped,
- 1tsp mixed herbs,
- 1 cup brown rice, cooked (2oz brown rice uncooked weight),
- Olive oil for cooking,

What you do with all this:
- Lightly fry the onion, garlic and mushrooms for about 10 minutes until the onions are transparent.
- Add the herbs and stir in the cooked brown rice. Add some freshly ground black pepper and stuff the mixture into the prepared peppers.
- Replace the top on the peppers and place them in an oven-proof dish. Bake for 20-30 minutes on gas mark 4.
- Serve with ratatouille or eat on their own.

Main Meals – Desserts

FAT OPTIONS	CARBOHYDRATE OPTIONS
- Sugar free ice cream (C, H, V) - Classic French chocolate mousse	- Berry compote (C, H, V) - Fruit puree (V)

Sugar Free Ice Cream (Serves 4)
You will need:
- Approximately 8oz or 200g of berries – strawberries, raspberries – whatever you fancy,
- 250ml double cream,
- 250ml Natural Live Yoghurt,
- An ice cream machine,

What you do with all this:
- Freeze the berries (remove any leaves or stalks first).
- Put the frozen berries into a blender with enough cream or yoghurt to cover them and start blending them. Once the frozen fruit is broken down, keep adding the rest of the yoghurt and cream until they are all blended in.
- Put the mixture in an ice-cream machine (follow the machine instructions) and then put it in the freezer once done.

You can make lots of variations to this recipe:
- Add more berries for a more fruity flavour,
- Add more yoghurt and less cream for a more tangy flavour,
- You can substitute fresh unsweetened orange juice for the yoghurt to make the recipe sweeter and more like a sorbet (Phase 3 only),
- You can add chopped frozen bananas to the recipe to make the consistency thicker (Phase 3 also).

(Please note that the next recipe for chocolate mousse and the one for mayonnaise contain raw eggs.)

Classic French Chocolate Mousse (Phase 3)

If you love chocolate this recipe is to die for. You can stand a spoon up in it and it will give you a chocolate high like you can't imagine. It is also as close to the rules of this book as chocolate can get as it is a fat meal in essence. Eat it at the end of a 'fat' dinner party and enjoy!

You will need:

- 8oz chocolate with at least 70% cocoa content (85% cocoa content makes the dessert even richer),
- 60ml of a cup of coffee (decaffeinated ideally),
- 2 large eggs – very fresh,
- 4 tablespoons sugar,
- 1 teaspoon vanilla extract,
- 2 tablespoons of dark rum,
- 240ml double cream (OK for whisking),
- An electric whisk,

What you do with all this:

- Separate the egg yolks and whites. Put the yolks in one mixing bowl and the whites in another.
- Using a hand held electric whisk beat the egg yolks until they are blended. Gradually add in 2 tablespoons of sugar, whilst blending all the time. Continue whisking for about 5 minutes or until the yolks turn pale yellow.
- Whisk in the rum and vanilla. Leave to one side for a moment.
- Break the chocolate bars into squares and put them into a saucepan with the liquid coffee. Stir together, over a low heat, until all the chocolate is melted.
- Add the melted chocolate and coffee to the egg yolks, rum and vanilla mixture. Leave to one side.
- Clean the whisk beaters thoroughly and then start to whisk the egg whites. Gradually add in the other 2 tablespoons of sugar to the egg whites and whisk the whole lot until stiff peaks form.
- Stir the egg white mixture gently into the mixture of egg yolk, rum, vanilla, chocolate and coffee.
- Using the empty egg white mixing bowl, whisk the cream until this is stiff and then add this to the other ingredients. Fold everything in together to mix it thoroughly and then pour and spoon the whole lot into a posh bowl ready for a dinner party.
- Place in the fridge and leave for at least 2 hours (it can be made the night before and left for 24 hours).

Berry Compote/Fruit Puree
You can use almost any fruit here, in almost any quantities. Experiment with different quantities of fruit in season to find the tastes that best suit you. Some of our favourites are: apples on their own; apple & blackberry; gooseberries or blackcurrants on their own. The berry compote is made by mixing any variation of berries – strawberries, raspberries and blackberries for example.

Chop the fruit and put it into a saucepan. Cook it slowly, with a small amount of water and with the lid on to preserve the juices, until the fruit has turned into a pulp. Be sure to stir regularly so that the fruit doesn't stick to the pan. Put a dollop onto your breakfast cereal or have it as a snack with Natural Live Yoghurt.

Extras

FAT OPTIONS	CARBOHYDRATE OPTIONS
- Mustard salad dressing (H, V)	- Ratatouille (C, H, V)
- Vinaigrette (H, V)	- Smoothies (V)
- Mayonnaise (C, H, P1, V)	

Extras – Fat options

Mustard Salad Dressing
Mix 3 teaspoons of mustard (any type without sugar) with 4-6 tablespoons of wine or cider vinegar, in a small container. Add 8-12 tablespoons of sunflower oil (there should always be twice as much oil as vinegar in salad dressings). Add some freshly ground black pepper and whisk, or shake, the mixture until smooth. This dressing can be kept in a sealed container in the fridge for up to three weeks. Be sure to shake well before each use.

Vinaigrette Salad Dressing
The basic recipe is to mix 2 measures of oil to 1 of vinegar and to mix thoroughly. Try the following variations:
- Olive oil and balsamic vinegar,
- Olive oil and cider vinegar (add a clove of crushed garlic and leave overnight for an added variation),
- Olive oil and lemon juice (great for fish dishes),
- Olive oil and fruit vinegar (e.g. raspberry).

Mayonnaise
This version is so easy to make and it is delicious. You need never buy mayonnaise from a shop again.
You will need:
- 1 egg yolk – very fresh,
- 2 tsp French mustard,
- Sunflower oil,
- Freshly ground black pepper,
What you do with all this:
- In a mixing bowl, vigorously whisk the egg yolk until smooth.
- Add the mustard and whisk some more. While continuing to whisk, slowly pour in the oil.
- Finally, add the pepper, give it a final whisk and serve.
Perfect mayonnaise in less than 2 minutes.

Extras – Carbohydrate options

Ratatouille (Serves 2)

This is great with fish or can be added to pasta instead of plain tomato sauce.

You will need:
- 2 courgettes/zucchini,
- 1 red pepper,
- 1 large onion (finely chopped),
- 1 clove garlic (finely chopped),
- 1 400g tin chopped tomatoes (check only tomatoes and citric acid are in the ingredients),
- Salt & Pepper,
- Olive oil for cooking,

What you do with all this:
- Chop the garlic and onions finely and then dice the courgettes/zucchini and pepper into slightly larger chunks.
- Heat a wok up until the olive oil is sizzling.
- Stir-fry the onion and garlic until slightly brown and then add the courgettes/zucchini, pepper and tomatoes.
- Add the salt & pepper and leave all to simmer until the vegetables are how you like them (some people like them on the verge of crunchy, others like them soft).

Smoothies

For all Smoothie recipes you should keep tubs full of frozen fruit in the freezer and then these fantastic drinks/desserts can be available within a couple of minutes at any time of the day. The base of all Smoothies is banana, so peel some ripe bananas (even slightly overripe is fine) and then chop them into slices no more than an inch thick and stick them in a tub in the freezer. For a variety of recipes you can also put a tub of raspberries in the freezer and strawberries (with the green hubs removed), blackberries and any other fruit you fancy. Please note that all Smoothies use fruit juice, which is refined fruit so Smoothies are a Phase 3 treat and they really are a treat. Give them to children at any time and see if they can tell that they have no sugar in them.

Strawberry and/or Raspberry Smoothie:

- Take a few pieces of frozen banana and put them at the bottom of a blender/liquidiser.
- Add some frozen strawberries and/or raspberries on top (play with the ratio to suit your taste – more banana will give a thicker texture; more strawberries will give more flavour. Start with an equal volume of each and then try different variations in the future).
- Pour unsweetened orange juice on top of the fruit to leave a few pieces sticking out above the liquid line. (Add in more juice if you are struggling to get it to blend).
- Turn the blender on. Shake the fruit around to get it nicely blended in.

Blackberry & Cranberry Smoothie:

- This is made in exactly the same way as the Strawberry recipe above except that you use blackberries instead of strawberries or raspberries and you use cranberry juice instead of orange juice.

Tropical Smoothie:

- This is made in exactly the same way as the Strawberry recipe above except that you use frozen mango or pineapple chunks instead of strawberries or raspberries and you use tropical fruit juice instead of orange juice.

TIP 1 – for a variation on all of the above you can add unsweetened Natural Live Yoghurt (NLY) in place of some of the juice. This gives a thick creamy texture and a bit of a tang – especially nice in the blackberry and cranberry Smoothie. If you add NLY to this Smoothie, you will be getting a double therapeutic blend of cranberry as a natural remedy for cystitis and NLY as a natural balance against Candida.

SEND IN A RECIPE...

Dear Reader,

Would you like one of your recipes included in our upcoming Recipe Book?
If so please complete the submission form overleaf (it can be torn out or photocopied) and send it with your recipe to:

Zoë Harcombe
PO Box 73
Caldicot
UK
NP26 3WD

We cannot guarantee to include all recipes but will let you know if we plan to use yours.

Please keep them healthy, simple and original!

THANK YOU

RECIPE SUBMISSION FORM

Name of recipe

....

How I'd like my name to appear in the book:

....

I now grant Zoë Harcombe a non-exclusive, royalty free, worldwide licence to print and publish this recipe.
I warrant that I am the sole owner of the copyright in the work and that I have full power to enter into this agreement.

Signed..

Name..

Email..

or

Address..

....

....

PLEASE PRINT CLEARLY IN INK.

RECIPES MUST BE ACCOMPANIED BY A FULLY COMPLETED SUBMISSION FORM IN ORDER TO BE CONSIDERED.

Thank you very much for reading

WHY DO YOU OVEREAT?
WHEN ALL YOU WANT IS TO BE SLIM

I can be contacted at
www.whydoyouovereat.com.

Zoë Harcombe